Naked Elbows

Naked Elbows

*A Physical Therapist's Reflections
on Patient Care, Intuition, and Healing*

Anne Ahlman, MPT

Gannett Healthcare Group

Gannett Healthcare Group
Division of Continuing Education
6400 Arlington Blvd., Suite 1000
Falls Church, VA 22042
ce@gannetthg.com
www.todayinpt.com

Cover photograph by Young Kim
Author photograph by Jim Ahlman

Printed and bound in the United States of America.

ISBN: 978-1-930745-05-6

Anne Ahlman's book *Naked Elbows* was generated from working in the trenches with thousands of patients with difficult physical therapy problems. Her insights demonstrate the art and skill of dealing comprehensively with an individual's varying condition, including their psychosocial well-being, pain tolerance, healing response, and capacity to handle adversity. These are valuable observations for all practitioners treating musculoskeletal problems.

Jeffrey S. Kliman, MD
Chief, Orthopaedic Surgery
El Camino Hospital
Mountain View, California

For my beloved husband, Jim

Contents

Foreword

Naked Elbows is an extremely delightful, humorous, and readable book, written professionally about a serious subject. The descriptions of day-to-day clinical situations were, for me, at times both touching and poignant, and at other times they made me laugh out loud. I experienced rueful recognition of the habits and behavior of both patients and members of my own health profession.

This is an unusual book for several reasons. It weaves the personal and professional into a rich tapestry, rather than being exclusively focused on one or the other. This provides a rainbow of color, which makes it anything but a dry book of case reports. Throughout the book, the author outlines her own journey toward the realization of a holistic approach to physical therapy, of the patient as the central focus, and of the practice of healing in general.

But it is also not just a collection of interesting experiences and observations. The book outlines the expanding scope of physical therapy, regarding both acute and chronic disease. Many preventive health messages that are applicable to everyone are embedded in the description of actual cases. This makes the book not only tremendously readable, but also important for practitioners, students, people undergoing physical therapy, and the general public.

Anne Ahlman's refreshing perspective is presented with an imaginative turn of phrase. The book has amplified my respect for the physical therapy profession, and has made me redouble my efforts at maintaining my own personal fitness and health. What better recommendation for a book?

Dr. Judith Longstaff Mackay
OBE, SBS, JP, MBChB (Edinburgh),
FRCP (Edinburgh), FRCP (London)
International Health Consultant

Preface

The stories that you are about to explore are true. This is a complete history and physical examination of my patients, my colleagues—and myself. No human interaction is ever truly one way, but is a mutual exchange of ideas and energy that flows between the participants. *Naked Elbows* is the first book to reveal the unique perspective of a practicing physical therapist on the human connection that occurs during individualized treatment. Because physical touch brings an immediate transference of energy and a sense of personal trust, within moments of a therapist's placing her hands on a patient she is transformed simultaneously into a bartender, confessor, and Mother Teresa.

This book is a reflection of how my efforts may have affected some of my patients, as well as how I have been touched by them in return. "Why didn't you become a doctor?" is a question I hear with regular frequency. Despite sharing with physicians a tendency toward appalling handwriting skills, I have never had any desire to become an MD. As a physical therapist, I am in the enviable position of being able to spend a lot of quality time with my patients, and am privileged to get to know them and share a portion of their lives as I help them make changes for the better.

To maintain patient confidentiality, in the following pages I have changed people's names but have retained the essence of our interactions together. Although I had originally intended to write this book to give people a glimpse into life from the clinician's side of the treatment table, I have found that the patients themselves often give me the greatest insight into the factors that contribute to healing. I am grateful to have formed such a profound connection with so many exceptional individuals as they willingly placed their broken bodies into my hands and their trust into my heart. Each person is so much more than the sum of his or her parts, and as a practicing physical therapist I attempt to treat each person as a valued family member whom I strive to listen to, care for, and learn from.

This book is dedicated to all of my patients but especially to Freddie and Larry, who endured some of my most enthusiastic treatment techniques yet who remain staunch supporters and good friends. The process of writing and publishing a book is similar to performing patient care in that it is part careful therapeutic progression and part hands-on mobilization, and I am indebted to the team at Gannett Healthcare Group for making it possible for me to reach my long-term goals. I owe particular thanks to Paul Murdock, PT, a wonderful clinician who welcomed my therapeutic talents and who gave me the space to write. Thank you also to Amanda J. S. Kaufmann for her true friendship, and to Stacey Lynn for her tactful suggestions and editorial wisdom, which enabled the manuscript to achieve functional independence.

My parents gave me a unique perspective on the world, but it is my mother's unwavering support and gifts of common sense and stoicism for which I am the most thankful. I am also deeply grateful to my special aunt Judith, a kindred spirit who has made all sorts of magical things possible in my life.

And to Jim—thank you for indulging my literary addiction, for bravely illuminating my path with good humor and infinite faith, and for giving me the best years of my life.

Anne Ahlman, MPT

Connecting with the Ninety Percent

You have something valuable. Every time I see Dr. K, he raves about you—you, especially. He says that you have a gift, a real talent for therapy.
—Freddie, intensive care unit nurse

I spend most of the day standing on my left leg. For some time, I had noticed a tendency to stand to the right of my bathroom sink so that I could center myself by leaning to the left when brushing my teeth. I also step into my left stirrup more forcefully when riding my horse (causing him to drift to the left over jumps) and sit harder on my left seat bone when charting, reading, or relaxing on the couch in front of the television set. One pivotal day, as I looked down at the square of flesh exposed between Anna's bra and waistband, I realized that my mobilizing hands on her back were placed several inches to the left of my body while I balanced easily on my left leg. I finally recognized that I always migrated to the left side of the treatment table in the clinic when mobilizing a patient's spine, and rested most of my weight on the left side whenever possible. How did I develop this habit? Why?

As a physical therapist, I am trained to look for imbalance and asymmetry in others but not necessarily within myself. This lopsided lean is a therapy-induced habit, one that is frowned upon by health professionals everywhere. I am chagrined to admit that I have allowed my habit to become entrenched ("But you're a physical therapist; you should know better!") and now spend much of my time reminding myself to stand and move with my weight more evenly distributed.

But for me the posture is valuable—it allows me to easily shift my weight away from my dominant arm, freeing my right hand for palpating, stretching, massaging, pushing, comforting, and patting my patients on the back.

~ ★ ~

Physicians say that 90 percent of the diagnosis lies within the patient history, and I have certainly found this to be true in the physical therapy clinic. When I first meet a patient, I sit quietly and simply ask, "So, what happened to you?" Usually, it all comes pouring out, and my greatest skill comes in redirecting the patient toward describing the current injury and away from that mysterious unrelated tumble from a wobbling bicycle at the tender age of six. However, I am careful to listen to the exact manner in which my patients describe their injuries, as they will unconsciously use the perfect words that give insight into their inner physical and emotional pain. During treatment, I am frequently entertained by spontaneous ramblings about the state of the world, the condition of the patient's personal relationships, and the location of the best local restaurants. Within this exchange of information live both the joys and the frustrations of the therapy experience.

It has been said that a good physical therapist is part Florence Nightingale and part Attila the Hun, and that it's up to the individual therapist to decide on the appropriate proportions. But physical therapy is more than just instructing patients to perform stretches and nagging them to do their exercises: it is a trusting personal connection that is deepened by the laying on of hands, the genuinely sympathetic touch, and the empowerment of progressively successful activity. This connection is augmented by the give and take of daily life. Everyone loves to hear a story, and this becomes especially useful to soothe and distract patients during the many uncomfortable moments when I must mobilize a painful joint or break down thickened scar tissue. As I help my patients unfurl their tight and battered bodies and heal their bruised souls, I exercise my storytelling skills and am honored by those who have chosen to share part of their lives with me in return. In the process of getting down to work, I roll up my sleeves, exposing both my naked elbows and my willingness to connect.

Part One

The Face

I think your whole life shows in your face and you should be proud of that.
—Lauren Bacall, American stage and screen actress (1924–)

If the eyes are the windows to the soul, then the face is the road map of each person's life experiences. When meeting new patients, I am always interested to observe their demeanor and facial expressions as they relate their histories to me. However, I must continually remind myself that they are checking me out with just as much alacrity, a fact that was brought home to me about ten years ago. I had entered the treatment room to meet an older patient who was in the clinic following her total hip replacement surgery when I saw her visibly relax and break into a relieved smile as soon as she saw my face. After we had introduced ourselves to each other, she blurted out, "I'm so glad you're not one of those *young* PTs!" For a moment I was nonplussed, but then accepted the compliment in the spirit in which it was given—I was glad that the sight of my experienced, slightly careworn features raised her confidence in my abilities. I have grown proud of my smile lines and feel I have earned all my wrinkles; consequently, I never hesitate to answer correctly when a patient asks me how old I am. Freddie, a retired intensive care unit nurse, patient, and friend commented that after a certain age you need to "choose between your face and your butt"; in other words, the face will become gaunt in our efforts to keep a trim posterior, yet maintaining enough body fat for a youthful face usually results in an exponential expansion of the rear end! Every day, I struggle to choose my butt.

Head Games

Life does not consist mainly, or even largely, of facts and happenings.
It consists mainly of the storm of thought that is forever flowing through one's head.
—Mark Twain, American humorist, writer, and lecturer (1835–1910)

The skin of the face is generally thinner than that in other areas of the body, and although it is richly supplied with nerves and blood vessels, the fragile tissues can become more susceptible to breakdown through habits of smoking or rubbing the delicate skin around the eyes in response to allergies. The many facial muscles are uniquely attached to the skull at one end and to other muscles or skin at the other end, unlike the majority of the body's muscles, which link bone to bone via tendons to enable movement. This anatomical arrangement of the facial muscles allows for a full range of emotional expression as we smile, frown, laugh, groan, and kiss. Sometimes this system can go awry despite our best intentions, as happened to my patient Jenny after her chin tuck surgery. Jenny had elected to have plastic surgery to "lift" her chin, but unfortunately her body's habit was to lay down a surprising amount of scar tissue following any sort of trauma, intentional or not. When I first saw her, she was unable to close her mouth to swallow without actively nodding her head toward her chest. It was only after a series of painful therapy sessions that included ultrasound and deep tissue mobilization to break down the scar tissue that she was able to voluntarily shut her jaw.

~ ★ ~

My father secretly wanted to be part of a traveling circus. He yearned to travel the world and take in every museum, castle, church, theater performance, and musical known to mankind. In hopes of achieving this ambition he got a job with Trans World Airlines, which gave him a generous vacation schedule and free term passes for the immediate family. My British mother was a willing fellow explorer, perhaps in part due to her own tumultuous childhood in which home was just a place to briefly touch the periphery of family life in wartime. During World War II, families throughout Britain were urged to evacuate their children to safety away from large population centers, which were thought to be more desirable targets for Hitler's bombs. Although my mother's home on the northeast coast of England was in a small Victorian seaside town, it was frequently bombed by fleeing Luftwaffe pilots as they sped back to Germany after failed sorties further inland. The town had two air raid shelters that were regularly unlocked to allow the inhabitants to spend safe but restless nights as the bombs dropped, but on one occasion, the warden was unable to locate the key for one of the shelters. Nearly the entire town huddled in the remaining shelter to endure yet another bombing run, and when they emerged after the all-clear signal, they found that the locked shelter had scored a direct hit. Fortunately, my mother was safely tucked into bed with her stuffed toy Scottie dog, miles away from the excitement, at boarding school.

My mother's childhood was spent living in relative safety away from the bosom of her family, with the pleasures of home life existing only as a half-remembered dream. Home was a place to become quietly regrounded before returning to the harsh reality of long terms spent away at school, and never seemed to be an achievable reality. Similarly, my childhood home in San Francisco seemed insubstantial and temporary; it was routine for my brother and I to jump onto an airplane at a moment's notice and fly virtually anywhere in the world at my parents' behest. Initially I took the gift of travel for granted, but over time I grew to dread particular trips at certain times of year.

One of the worst such journeys always began with my father bundling us onto a last-minute red-eye flight to New York City over the holidays. We would stagger directly onto the airplane from the crew bus in the dead of night, tiredly read novels or play travel chess as the plane churned eastward, and then disembark to ride the bus into the city only to stand in line for tickets to the Christmas show at Radio City Music Hall. It was always bitterly cold, and despite our attempts to cheer ourselves up with warm roasted chestnuts from the omnipresent street vendors, we shivered inside our inadequate polyester California clothes, our faces mottled pink with cold. When we eventually shuffled to the front of the huge line and made it into the plush hall, we'd sleep through the first show sprawled across the theater seats in toasty splendor, watch the second show, and then fly home again the same day. I much preferred to travel to England to visit my beloved maternal family, where the countryside was picturesque and peaceful despite similarly cool temperatures. My grandmother's house in North Yorkshire always felt like my true home, where roots could be nurtured and the soul restored, and I resented having to return to the chilly, seemingly inhospitable City by the Bay after such idyllic times.

Since I am not blessed with a strong vestibular system and usually suffered from motion sickness whenever we left home, my general dislike of travel was compounded. However, suffering from this uncomfortable and sometimes embarrassing malady prompted me to choose vestibular exercise therapy for the topic of my master's thesis in an effort to learn more about the disorder that had plagued me so relentlessly throughout my early years.

The idea of vestibular rehabilitation is to influence the inner ear, which serves as an internal reference of where our head is in space in relation to our bodies, in conjunction with the visual and somatosensory systems. When someone suffers from vestibular dysfunction there is a conflict between these systems; it is this conflict that promotes the feeling of clamminess and eventual nausea and vomiting. Therapy is often based on accommodation of the inner ear by a series of supervised and then independent home exercises that stimulate eye, head, neck, and body positions. This type of therapy is similar to the experience of landlubbers who first take to the high seas—after several days of revolting illness and incapacitation, in most cases the disconnected vestibular system finally accommodates to the motion of the ship and allows the horrendous symptoms to dissipate.

~ ★ ~

One of my first encounters with a vestibular patient other than myself occurred while I was still in physical therapy (PT) school. The patient, Ben, had been working with my professor and mentor for one or two sessions on the treadmill, as in his case the conflict of stimuli brought about by running on a moving surface while not actually going anywhere would bring on dizziness—there was a disconnect between what his body (somatosensory system), his eyes (visual system), and his inner ear (vestibular system) were telling him. I had personally experienced and also learned in school that the symptoms typically experienced by vestibular patients were dizziness, imbalance, and nausea, so I thought I knew what to expect. But, when my instructor left the room, Ben began to explain his distressing symptoms in greater detail. "I've noticed that if I close my eyes while I'm standing or walking, I fall over. I want to be able to run on the treadmill during the winter, but after about five or ten minutes I start to feel a tingling sensation in my face! It feels really weird, as if I'm about to have an orgasm."

I shot a suspicious look at Ben to see if he was pulling my leg—was this some kind of strange joke? Or was he one of those weird guys who just loved to get a reaction from girls? However, Ben was serious. "I mean, I don't mind the feeling; in fact, it's kind of pleasurable, but it builds up so strongly I start getting dizzy and then I have to quit running." Before I had the chance to respond, my instructor returned and started working with Ben as he walked on the treadmill, performing a variety of vestibular exercises, while I observed. Later, I found out that this type of facial tingling feeling can occur in cases of an underlying acoustic neuroma, a benign tumor of the eighth cranial nerve (the vestibulocochlear nerve), which is responsible for hearing and balance. I was grateful to realize that this was truly a physical, not a psychological, condition.

~ ★ ~

During my time in graduate school at the joint program in physical therapy offered by the University of California at San Francisco and San Francisco State University (UCSF/SFSU), guest experts arrived from time to time to impart their knowledge to our blossoming group of PT students. At that time we were in awe of PTs with even five years of experience (oh, to be so confident!) and set the international experts firmly onto pedestals of fawning adoration. One such expert from Hawai'i, Andrew, visited us to share his special perspective on the intricacies and anomalies of human anatomy, and on temperomandibular joint (TMJ) disorder in particular. The temperomandibular joints are the connections between the skull and the lower jaw (mandible) that allow us to open and close our mouths, chew, yell, and sing. The joint surfaces are separated by articular discs, with the gliding motion of the joints easily palpated by gently placing the fingertips into the patient's ears as they slowly open and close the jaw. Standing at the front of our cadaver lab, Andrew began with a brief review of TMJ disorders and upper cervical spine anatomy before turning his attention to one of our patiently waiting cadavers.

Although gross anatomy is a prerequisite course for the PT school application process, most undergraduate cadaver labs consist of one cadaver per thirty to fifty students or more. Since there wasn't enough body surface area for all of us to gain access to the corpse at once, we weren't allowed to actively dissect our own cadavers but instead were taken on guided tours of previously dissected cadavers by the instructor. I privately suspected that part of the reason that we had to retain a passive, observational role was to cut down on the number of fainting episodes that regularly occurred each year.

The cadaver labs were initially frightening, then fascinating. We were shown the most personal parts of the body in intimate detail, and any disgust that we felt quickly turned into frowns of concentration as we struggled with the Latin names of all the little bits and pieces. We were eventually tested on our memory capacity via the dreaded lab practical. Lab practical examinations were given in a room overflowing with trays of dismembered body parts that were strewn about on every available surface. Each tray contained a random arm or foot with little flags stuck into specific parts of it; we were required to identify the anatomical landmark (muscle, tendon, ligament, nerve) that corresponded to the tip of the flagged pin. Other practical stations involved X-rays of a spine or a pelvis, microscope slides with smears of muscle cells, and plastic skeletons tagged at bony landmarks. (Question: Which large respiratory muscle is innervated by the nerve roots of the third, fourth, and fifth cervical [C] vertebrae? Answer: C3, 4, and 5 keep the diaphragm alive). The overwhelming atmosphere of the anatomy lab was that of revulsion to the strong formaldehyde odors, fascination at seeing how much the nerves really do look like strands of linguine, and resolution to not disgrace ourselves by passing out when faced with a real human uterus in situ.

We were fortunate to have a shrouded roomful of whole cadavers at our disposal in the huge lab overlooking Golden Gate Park at UCSF, as well as assorted body parts, brains, and bones to work with. Here we were assigned to our own cadavers according to last name, in alphabetical order, with one aromatically preserved corpse allotted to every four students. The first time I peeled back the draping sheet I was prepared for flight, but fortunately the cadaver's head was securely bound into a cheesecloth pillowcase and I couldn't directly see his face. Instead, I could make out a faded, spreading greenish-black tattoo of a rooster etched onto a large right deltoid—apparently, our muscular man had been a longshoreman in his youth.

We were instructed to dissect the muscles along the back in an attempt to ease us gently into the horror of actually cutting into a person. At first we stood around self-consciously looking at each other (you go first—no, *you*), until I screwed up my courage and grabbed a sharp scalpel, plunging it into the cadaver's back with a grimace. Once the first cut was done the worst was over, and with time I forgot my fears as I became hardened to the violent sights and smells and began to see it all as straightforward, simple anatomy. Despite the eventually routine nature of exploring the body's mysteries, the one thing I never forgot was that this person beneath me had once been a valued member of someone's family, an individual who had loved, laughed, made mistakes and been forgiven, and who chose to sacrifice a traditional burial or cremation in order to let medical students "see."

The day Andrew came to discuss the finer points of TMJ anatomy, he chose a cadaver from another group's table to work with. As his talk was being filmed, Andrew dissected the muscles of the jaw and described the intricate machinations that occurred during mastication. Then, he decided to expose the upper cervical spinal anatomy to demonstrate the close association between the muscles of the jaw and the upper neck. The film rolled smoothly on as Andrew worked to free the upper cervical muscles and tendons from superficial to deep as he discussed the many layers. Then, he chose to release the head from the neck to more intimately display the temperomandibular joints from beneath. He gestured to two nearby PT students and instructed, "You two, at the feet—hold tight! I will now pull the head away . . ." as he grasped the cadaver's head and leaned back in a waterskiing position, pulling with all his strength. The camera wobbled slightly as the cameraman nervously shifted his feet.

"OK, this should come away more easily. How old is this guy? Maybe the ligaments have ossified." Andrew continued to tug at the cadaver's head in a series of strong jerks, sweat pouring down his face. The class shifted apprehensively, and I sneaked another look at the cameraman. He was swiftly turning gray as the camera began to tremble in his shaking hands. The students at the cadaver's feet braced themselves . . . and with a loud crack the head came off into Andrew's lap, forcing him to unexpectedly sit down on the laboratory floor with an air of mild surprise. The camera continued filming the empty doorway at a rakish angle as it lay sideways on the lab stool, rocking slightly—the cameraman could take no more.

~ ★ ~

I glanced down at the new chart containing the physician's referral stating "TMJ—Evaluate and Treat," and gently knocked on the door of treatment room number five. When I pushed it open, I found an attractive dark-haired woman in her late twenties flipping rigidly through a magazine, barely glancing at the pages. Her jaw was clenched, and as she looked up at me she impatiently pushed her cat's-eye style glasses farther up onto her nose. Then, she leapt off the treatment table where she had been waiting and grabbed my right hand, pumping it vigorously. "I'm so pleased to meet you. I hope you can help; I'm at my wits' end! I've seen a ton of doctors and therapists, and no one seems able to get to the bottom of my problem."

My heart sank. What could I possibly do for her that hadn't already been done? We began to comb through her history, and I found that Nancy had seen a dentist, a craniofacial specialist, and a neurologist. She had undergone X-rays and diagnostic ultrasounds, and had received physical therapy before at a different clinic for her chronic intermittent jaw pain. She had been prescribed an array of medications including anti-inflammatories, painkillers, and even narcotics. But, the pain in her right jaw remained, waking her in the night and disturbing her concentration during the day.

As I began to examine Nancy, I could find nothing obviously wrong with her neck or jaw movement. She had a normal amount of jaw opening with no apparent deviation to either side, and no increased pain when clenching her jaw. She did mention that sometimes she could taste something "funny" in her mouth, but was unable to identify what the flavor was or what would trigger the sensation. I invited her to lie down on the treatment table, explaining that I wanted to palpate the muscles around her upper neck and jaw. As she lay prone, I felt for restrictions in the upper cervical vertebrae and found slightly increased stiffness in response to gentle mobilization of the right C1 and C2 vertebral transverse processes. Then, I asked Nancy to turn over so that I could palpate the muscles around her face and jaw in supine. As I looked down at her face from above, I could see that her face was more rounded on the right than on the left. I asked, "Have you ever noticed swelling in your face? It looks like your right cheek sticks out a little further than the left one." Nancy sat bolt upright, craning around to stare at me. "I thought that was all in my head! I could swear the right side of my face feels swollen sometimes, but no one has ever been able to see it." I reassured her that I could see it only from my vantage point of looking down at her upside-down face, but it was most definitely there.

Nancy resumed her supine position and I proceeded to gently apply moisturizing lotion to her cheeks, explaining that the lotion would cut down on skin friction and enable me to feel the deeper muscles and soft tissues of her face and jaw. She looked up at me, perplexed. "No one has ever done that before." Now it was my turn for confusion. "You mean that no one has ever felt your jaw muscles for lumps and bumps? However did you get the diagnosis of 'TMJ'?" Nancy shrugged, and said matter-of-factly, "No one really knows what's wrong with me."

As I palpated her cheeks simultaneously with the fingertips of both hands, I discovered that not only was her right masseter jaw muscle enlarged and hypertonic, but within the muscle were three tiny hard lumps. As I gently probed the lumps, Nancy winced. "That's the pain. What is that?" I was at a complete loss. Suddenly, I had a mental image of my horse champing at his bit—when horses are correctly ridden "on the bit," the angle of the head on the neck is such that they generate large amounts of white, frothy saliva from their parotid (salivary) glands. Slowly, I replied, "I think you might have a problem with the salivary glands in your cheek. Is the pain worse when you eat? Do you feel like you have dryness in your mouth? This can happen if there are stones in the gland that actually block the flow of saliva into your mouth."

Nancy agreed that she had been experiencing dry mouth, but thought that this was just a side effect of the medications she had been trying. I could not explain why, if there were stones lodged somewhere in the salivary gland or duct, they did not show up on her previous X-rays, since stones are typically composed of calcium. (Later, I found out that only approximately 15 percent of parotid gland stones are visible on X-ray). However, I showed Nancy how to relax her tight jaw muscles with self-massage and warm compresses, and urged her to revisit her physician for further tests to help confirm my suspicions. We eventually discovered that Nancy did indeed have salivary gland stones that were large enough to require surgical removal, solving her problem.

~ ★ ~

It takes a lot of time and practice to develop the kind of "feel" in your fingertips that lets you see without using your eyes. In addition, patient care itself can take quite some getting used to. In PT school there is a progressive, gradual immersion into the physical and psychological approaches to handling patients. At first, you learn by practicing on your fellow students. In this way you can experience all the surprisingly difficult methods by which you handle limbs, palpate soft tissues, and mobilize spines. Then, you learn how to take blood pressure readings and pulses, how to read the plastic goniometer when measuring the angles associated with joint range of motion, and how to carefully wield the sinister-looking "pizza cutter" tool that is gently used to search for changes in skin sensation.

My class of thirty PT students was reduced to mass hysteria when we learned how to find deep tendon reflexes. We spent hours practicing the correct way to bang the little red rubber-tipped hammer on each other's prominent tendons to produce the desired knee- or ankle-jerk response, and the women often ran home giggling at the end of the day to try out the mysterious cremasteric reflex on their unsuspecting boyfriends and husbands. This reflex can be elicited by stroking the inner, upper thigh with the tip of the reflex hammer handle, which results in a drawing-up of the ipsilateral scrotum in males; the absence of this response can demonstrate problems with the first and second lumbar nerve roots and may also indicate testicular torsion.

After passing numerous lab practical examinations in which we nervously demonstrated our newly discovered skills on our PT instructors, we were finally introduced to real patients. During my time spent working on my master's degree at UCSF/SFSU, I found that those patients were the true experts. Culled from failed physical therapy sessions over at the main hospital, these patients had some of the most challenging conditions known in the clinic. The patients had seen it all, and were extremely generous of spirit in allowing us to touch them with our mediocre, fumbling, self-conscious fingers. Sometimes they would whisper "test my anterior tibialis muscle—it's denervated" when the instructor wasn't looking during a lab practical in an effort to point us in the right direction during a diagnostic workup. Although physically handling each patient seemed demanding at first, the logistics of positioning limbs and performing tests soon became matter-of-fact and my confidence grew. However, it would take a lot more experience to learn my way around the inner patient.

~ ★ ~

The path to creating a good bedside manner begins with projecting your interest, sincerity, compassion, and undivided attention toward the patient. Being an active listener is essential, a skill that developed early for me. I have always felt a tremendous drive to be helpful to others. When I played as a child, I usually had one ear listening for my parents' whereabouts, ready to respond if they needed anything. Despite my innate yearnings to smooth the furrowed brows of everybody around me, I often suffered from what my family called "drawbridge syndrome"—the tendency to withdraw into oneself. In other words, once I was in my "castle" for the day, I would pull up the imaginary drawbridge, release the pretend alligators into the moat, and relax in solitary peace and tranquility. Over the years my personal castle became much more than just our physical house, and transcended my entire self. Whereas I enjoyed the company of other people (especially if I could do something for them), I was a classic introvert who regenerated her energy in solitude. This approach worked well until I discovered that my face did not reflect my inner peace when in repose. Somehow, I needed to work on my outward affect if I wanted my patients to feel welcome and safe with me.

"You always look so serious!" my friends would exclaim in concern. Even my husband enquired, "Is everything alright?" with exhausting regularity. But it didn't stop there. "Man, you're really hostile," strangers would comment as I strode past them in my own little world, projecting my default protect-yourself-by-looking-confident-in-the-city mode. What was wrong with everyone? I was just relaxed, thinking my thoughts, safe inside the inner castle within my head.

Then, I caught pneumonia for the first time. It was serious enough that it prevented my going out to work, but during my recovery I found that I could prop myself up in bed on a frothy sea of pillows to work on my writing on the laptop computer. Usually I am able to focus with single-minded concentration regardless of my surroundings—noisy airports, booming television programs, and screaming children fade to a faint buzzing sound in my ears—but in the aftermath of my lung infection I was easily distracted. And so it was that one day in the midst of my recovery, I looked up and caught sight of myself. There it was. My scowling face, reflected in the beveled mirror in the armoire facing our bed. But I was just thinking! How stern I looked; it was no wonder I received the feedback that I did. As I thought about the problem, my frown deepened and I inwardly winced. I remembered mentally accusing a PT colleague of being aloof and egocentric until our paths had crossed and I had finally gotten to know her. Carly was very attractive, with beautiful olive skin, large brown eyes, long well-groomed mahogany hair, and a sense of style, but she seemed distant and "stuck up" (a quality I had frequently been labeled with over the years). It turned out that she had a reserved expression only when she was walking around by herself or when she concentrated on documenting her SOAP (subjective, objective, assessment, and plan) notes in the patient charts. But in fact her smile was like sunshine on autumn leaves and her laugh was explosive in its wholeheartedness. Carly and I ended up being great friends after our initial meeting at a staff function, when she confessed that she had thought me unapproachable too.

As I continued to absently consider my stern reflection as it glared back at me, I remembered another embarrassing time when a patient complained to the clinic manager that I "didn't say hello" to her as I walked through the lobby to put away my belongings before starting the workday. At the time I was deeply affronted; after all, was I supposed to walk around with a grin like a village idiot plastered on my face? I had always made an effort to put people at their ease—humph. But, I conceded now, at the time I had no idea just how dour my expression actually appeared when I was deep in thought. I realized that in the past my only saving grace had been the trust-inspiring clear gaze of my light blue-gray eyes, combined with my eager response to assist others. But now I could use my newfound self-awareness to help permanently etch the smile lines onto my face. I practiced a little in the armoire mirror; no, that was a grimace. Another effort—even worse, it looked like I was apologetically passing gas. After many minutes amusing myself with all manner of grotesque expressions, I finally tried looking away as I thought about my husband and pets—there. A pleasant, gentle smile had appeared. Success! It was simply a matter of projecting my inner compassion and my desire to please upon my outer visage. Clearly, I would need more practice.

~ ★ ~

In the process of developing my skills as a physical therapist, I felt that I needed to experience all aspects of the therapeutic environment. One of my favorite areas of practice is geriatrics, as I had been raised to have a healthy respect for my elders and had enjoyed a special relationship with my maternal grandmother, who had been ahead of her time—she was one of the first women in England to attend university. Granny was born in 1905 during Edwardian times, and her life traversed the coronation of five kings and queens of England, the deprivations of World War I, the rationing of World War II, and the triumphant return of my grandfather, her brave naval captain husband, who gallantly brought his crew to safety after being torpedoed by a Nazi U-boat. Granny died gracefully on her ninety-fifth birthday after revisiting our family photos for the last time and having a bite of her birthday cake with a few sips of her favorite dry white wine. Throughout her life, Granny remained an incredible source of history, faith, and humor, and was a beacon of integrity and strength for the entire family—a true matriarch. My family sentiment, combined with a natural affinity for the wisdom and storytelling abilities of the elderly, led me to work in the environment of nursing homes for a number of years.

Society seems to assume that the elderly just don't feel pain in the same way their younger counterparts do, but as we get older we become more skilled about hiding our emotions and pain responses for the sake of others. We have "seen it all before," weathered many storms, and become increasingly stoic in the face of adversity. I have discovered that I can never truly know what is going on inside someone else's head; it is difficult enough sorting out my own feelings and emotions, let alone trying to fully grasp someone else's problems. In the nursing home setting, physical therapy can be enormously rewarding and frustrating all at once as therapists try to deal with the combined histories of centuries, occasionally stained with the overlap of dementia.

Perception is uniquely our own, and nowhere have I seen this more acutely than in the setting of an Alzheimer's unit. One of the convalescent hospitals I worked in for several years had a short-term Medicare wing for treatment of patients who might go home again after their rehabilitation, several long-term care sections for patients who needed additional help in order to survive, an unlocked Alzheimer's unit for demented patients too far along to move independently anymore, and a locked Alzheimer's unit for those who were at risk to wander away in their confusion and possibly get lost or hurt. As the lead physical therapist and eventually director of rehabilitation at the facility, I had intimate involvement in all four settings. However, the locked unit was a constant source of awe and learning, teaching me that we truly do live inside our own heads, especially when we are unable to reach out to others.

No two people are affected by Alzheimer's disease in the exact same way, perhaps because no two people are alike to begin with. All individuals have their own personal and family history, current relationships, inner emotions, and hopes and fears that set them apart. At first, the signs of oncoming dementia can be terrifying when a patient begins to realize that her mind is patchily fading; after all, who hasn't had a brief moment of panic when an ATM code or the location of a parked car is momentarily forgotten? But, as the mind slips further into dementia, the patient moves beyond self-awareness and lives in a twilight consisting of past memories and current moment-by-moment reactions. These are the years that are hardest on the family, when the patient only has random glimpses of what went before. In response, some family members withdraw from the emotional pain of not being remembered and stop visiting the patient, while others become more involved by bringing daily changes of clothing, reading to the patient, or simply helping to feed them. Some patients with Alzheimer's disease can become anxious, paranoid, or combative, while others purposefully wander the hallways searching for a familiar sight to guide them back home. As brain function declines even further, patients stop wandering and eventually forget how to walk, stand, sit up, and even swallow without help.

Chester, a patient with Alzheimer's disease who was no longer able to speak and who required the help of two nurses to get in and out of bed, was one of the residents in the unlocked unit—poor Chester was simply not mobile enough to try to find his way home again. Chester's daughter visited him every day without fail and helped him eat lunch, since he would take in a higher percentage of his meal in her vaguely familiar presence. In her efforts to make his stay pleasant and homelike, she constructed a memory book of family photos to place on his bedside table and hung soothing seaside pictures on the adjacent wall, where he could see and touch them from his bed. She began to notice, however, that Chester kept tearing down her pictures of seahorses, waves, and shells. With hurt feelings, she stopped me in the hallway one day and asked if I could help her figure out what was wrong with Chester. "I just don't understand it," she said. "You would think these beach pictures would help him feel calmer and more relaxed. But every time I come in here, I can see where he's been clawing them off the walls!"

"Is the seaside a familiar, comforting place for him?" I asked. "Does he have fond memories of childhood vacations at the shore, or is he drawn to the sea in some way?"

She paused to reflect. "Not really, I guess—he grew up on a farm in the Midwest, and was into horse-drawn machinery in his youth, come to think of it!" she replied.

"Why don't you try putting up pictures of crops and fields, or horses pulling a plow?" I suggested.

The next time I passed Chester's room a few days later, I saw that his daughter had been busy. Fastened to the walls around his bed were scenes of peacefully grazing horses, and across from his bed hung a picture of the sun setting over fields of corn on a glorious midsummer day. Chester himself was lying contentedly in bed, gazing at the horses that grazed calmly on the wall nearby. Life has little meaning outside of the context of its relationships, and Chester was finally at peace with the surroundings that made him feel at home.

~ ★ ~

Certain patients with Alzheimer's disease have gotten inside my skin and delivered blows to my own perception of reality. I worked with Louise after she had fallen and broken her arm when she climbed over her raised bedrails; she needed PT because she had forgotten how to walk while wearing the arm sling that stabilized her healing bones. Louise loved to talk, and would happily carry on both sides of the conversation during the entire treatment session, mostly reliving her childhood with her three sisters in Italy. Throughout our one-sided conversation, I would have to interrupt her briefly to cue her to shift her weight, come from sit to stand, or hold onto the railing along the hallway wall as she relearned how to ambulate. Undeterred, Louise would smoothly follow my directions without disrupting her story. On certain days she was calmer and I could ask her questions about Italy and her childhood home, but on others she was unable to remember anything and would be combative and agitated. One day, Louise was especially feisty and was railing on about her sisters' behavior at Mass "that morning." In my effort to distract her and reduce her agitation, I entered her world and asked, "What are your sisters doing now? Are they making lunch for you while we chat, or have they gone out to the market?" Louise stopped walking, looked at me pityingly, and in a moment of clarity said, "Oh, them—all three of them have Alzheimer's, can you believe it? Poor fools, they wouldn't remember how to boil pasta if they tried."

~ ★ ~

The unlocked part of the hospital was disturbing at times, but the locked part was entirely surreal. This part of the building was built as a square around an inner courtyard, so patients could keep moving if they wished without encountering a frustratingly locked door in their paths. Some patients would pace the halls in the same direction all day long, as if they were inside a giant fish roundabout, while others would meander from room to room, absentmindedly picking up a sock or hairbrush and then walking on, occasionally colliding with the more focused characters. Scuffles broke out frequently, and certain patients could become violent if you looked at them with the wrong expression. However, most of the patients responded to a smile and a kind word, and those who didn't were given medication to prevent them from becoming so agitated that they might hurt themselves or others. Symptoms of agitation, increased confusion, and anxiety typically worsen toward evening; a recognized phenomenon called "sundowning." As the sun sets, the agitation rises. Sundowning occurs in up to 20 percent of patients with Alzheimer's, especially during the middle stages of the disease's progression.

A few of the patients who were confirmed wanderers in the locked facility would fall from time to time. Some, like Philip, were quite adventurous; somehow, he once managed to climb onto the roof of the facility, forcing us to clamber up after him and coax him safely down. Many were less adventurous souls who were silently trying to seek comfort and familiarity. Kevin, a special patient who had maintained a sweet demeanor throughout his decline into dementia, would spend hours sorting through blank papers at the nursing station to fulfill his self-appointed obligation to his clients—in better days he had been a lawyer, and he was accustomed to handling briefs. This minor act kept him happily fulfilled and occupied and made him feel useful. Marie, a native New Yorker, took delight in brushing her teeth and then whipping out into the hallway wearing only her nightgown, her mouth foaming with toothpaste and her eyes twinkling as she exclaimed, "Look—mad dog, Mad Dog!"

But one day a quiet, rather introverted patient named Peter, who normally just drifted slowly around the halls, lost his balance in a scuffle with Philip and broke his hip. When this happens to a person with severe dementia, the orthopedic surgeon has a difficult decision to make: if the hip is surgically replaced, the patient may inadvertently dislocate the new hip because he is simply unable to remember the standard total hip precautions not to bend the hip more than 90 degrees, cross the legs, or internally rotate the limb. However, if the hip is pinned (open reduction with internal fixation), there is a healing period during which time the patient is not allowed to fully bear weight on the leg until the bone has begun to strengthen around the repair. Of course, the patient with dementia can't remember not to stand on the leg with his full weight, so recovery is fraught with peril.

Peter's surgeon decided to replace the hip, since it was too damaged at the femoral head to pin; plus, with Peter's tendency to wander, he was unknowingly putting himself at risk for overloading a pinned hip before it was ready to bear his weight. My role was to help Peter safely get back up on his feet, no easy task following anesthesia for someone with dementia; typically, anesthesia will transiently make the dementia worse. For his immediate recovery period, Peter was admitted into the short-term Medicare wing so that I could work with him twice a day and so he could receive specialized postsurgical care. For the time being, because he had forgotten how to walk, Peter was no longer a wandering risk. Each day Peter became physically stronger and more like his old self, and we developed an easy working relationship. Although Peter initially needed the help of parallel bars and then a walker to lean on, his balance steadily improved. As he became more independent, the nursing staff began to get nervous that Peter might try to walk on his own and possibly leave the building unknowingly, and started to discuss the timing of sending him back to the locked unit.

One fine spring morning, Peter had walked especially well with me but was tired and wanted to lie down for awhile to take a nap before lunch. I helped him back to his bed, got him comfortably arranged with his protective adductor pillow between his knees to prevent him accidentally crossing his legs, and made sure that his call light was nearby in case he remembered how to use it. As I turned the light out in his room and asked him if I could get anything else for him before I left, Peter looked at me with a lucid, knowing smile and told me, "I'm going home this afternoon." I racked my brain as to what he meant. In the morning facility Stand-up Meeting there had been no mention of his returning to live with his family. Did he mean he was going back to the locked facility later that day? I decided to check on my way out to lunch.

"That's great!" I said with an encouraging smile. "It'll be so nice for you to be home again. Are you looking forward to it, or will you miss us too much over here?" I teased.

"Yeah, I'll miss you a little," he conceded, "but I can hardly wait to get home again." He shut his eyes decisively, and I left him to his nap.

When I returned after lunch, all the nurses were talking: "Did you hear about Peter? I can't believe he's dead! So sudden!" Peter had somehow indeed known where he was going and had quietly drifted off after I left him. He had found his way Home.

~ ★ ~

"I'm going to order a turducken this weekend to give my fiancé for Christmas," my preceptor Terry confided to me merrily as we made our way toward our first patient of the day.

"Who, or what, is a turducken?" I asked quizzically, my apprehension about meeting our new patient with a diagnosis of "Head Injury—Evaluate and Treat" momentarily stilled.

"A turducken is a turkey, stuffed with a duck, which is then stuffed with a chicken. Greg says he has always wanted one, so I thought I'd surprise him this year!" Terry responded with a laugh.

"Oh—OK. It sounds like the tryptophan content should knock him out through the end of the year. Now, what's the scoop on this new patient?" I anxiously redirected.

As a second year PT student, I was now in the midst of a clinical rotation at an inpatient neuro rehab center and was finding it difficult. When I had first applied to PT school, I was confident that I would love neurology, since central nervous system injuries could be approached in a multitude of different ways to help patients improve and compensate for their deficits. Initially, the plasticity and pliability of the human brain and nervous system had intrigued me after watching my newly retired father rapidly recover from a small stroke. But after struggling through my neuroanatomy coursework and meeting patients who had suffered spinal cord injuries and massive strokes, I was rapidly becoming less enthusiastic. What had at first seemed merely interesting and creative to deal with now seemed impossible to grasp—I just couldn't seem to see what to do, nor summon any intuition about how to handle these patients. I found myself wishing for the relatively concrete world of orthopedics for the thousandth time.

"Duane is a twenty-one-year-old gunshot wound to the head," said Terry, consulting the chart. "He had a successful surgery to remove the bullet, but the damage has left him without the ability to stand or walk. In fact, it looks like he can't even transfer yet from bed to wheelchair without being totally dependent on help because his balance is so poor. Oh, the good news is that he has spasticity, so if we play our cards right we can get him to 'walk on his tone.' Let's see . . . hmm, hmm . . . looks like he has some 'inappropriate behavior' too, probably since the bullet destroyed part of his limbic system. Let's go meet him!"

We knocked and entered the treatment room and encountered a tall, dark-haired boy strapped into a wheelchair, with a vest restraint and a lap tray positioned to keep him from sliding out or tipping over. The occupational therapist had already worked with him to get him dressed and sitting up, and he was attired in loose-fitting athletic snap-on sweatpants and a T-shirt. Although one side of his face appeared completely normal, he was apparently unconscious that there was a line of saliva slowly dribbling from the opposite side of his mouth. Duane did not look up at us or acknowledge our presence in any way, but was transfixed on an imaginary point in the middle distance as his right hand explored his crotch, inside his underwear. The left hand was curled at the end of a rigid upper extremity that was flexed protectively in front of his body, hovering above the lap tray as he leaned toward the left.

Terry and I exchanged looks, and began unpacking Duane from his restraints. "Hi, Duane, we're going to help you get back on your feet," chirped Terry as we worked to free him from his bonds. "Let's wheel him over to the treatment mat and see if we can work on some transfer training," she suggested to me. "OK, Duane, put that away! Let's get moving." After a great deal of verbal cueing and facilitative hand pressures, we were able to transfer him from his wheelchair to seat him on the edge of the mat using a slide board. Immediately, Duane began to push himself toward his weak left side, and nearly fell over. Inwardly, I groaned—he was a pusher.

Pusher syndrome, a frustrating condition that can occur with damage to the brain from a variety of traumas, gives patients the false perception that their bodies are tilting to the side in relation to gravity. Of course, they naturally try to push themselves back to an "upright" position; unfortunately, this compensatory response results in them pushing themselves over toward the affected side when sitting or standing, an action that often ends in a fall. One of the treatment methods to help solve the problem is to work with patients during sitting, standing, and walking activities as they are able while helping them focus on their visual surroundings; somehow, through visual feedback and weight shifting exercises, patients can be guided into an erect position with the strategic use of mirrors and cues to help them see and feel when they are leaning over.

We arranged the treatment mirror so that Duane could see his reflection easily. Although he had continued to remain silent, he was clearly captivated by his appearance in the mirror and immediately tried to lift his chest and straighten up. Encouraged, we worked on a variety of exercises with him to challenge his sitting balance and reinforce the upright position. As we worked, we noticed a curious phenomenon in that he kept gradually trying to scoot to the left. I kneeled behind him on the treatment mat to see if I could understand why he was doing this, and noticed that by shifting over he was no longer able to see the damaged left side of his face and body in the mirror. This realization twisted my heart—here was a young, athletic guy in his prime, but with an extremely uncertain prognosis for returning to his old way of life.

By the end of the treatment session, Duane was able to scoot to and from the wheelchair and the treatment mat using the slide board as long as we guided him along the board and held onto his long trunk with a gait belt so that he wouldn't inadvertently nose dive onto the floor. Despite his lack of ability to outwardly communicate, Duane was clearly receiving visual and verbal input from the mirror and from us. As I knelt there behind him looking into our mirrored right halves, I noticed an unseen tear slowly form and trickle down the left side of his handsome face. Over many treatments, we were able to help Duane stop pushing and to stand and walk again with minimal assistance to help his tall frame maintain its balance, but he was never to regain an independent lifestyle. Neuro rehab represented great sadness to me after that, and I subsequently gravitated toward the more logical, mechanical world of orthopedics.

~ ★ ~

Despite my building disillusionment with neurology, I kept my hand in with special neurological cases in a less formal setting after I graduated from PT school. I had discovered hippotherapy when I was a student, a treatment technique that seemed like the perfect match between two of my great interests—horses and physical therapy. Hippotherapy literally means "treatment with the help of the horse" and involves using the dynamic platform of a horse's back to challenge all sorts of bodily systems. At that time the majority of our clients were children with developmental delay or neurological deficits from conditions such as cerebral palsy. Some were unable to hold up their own heads, others could not communicate, and still others were confined to a wheelchair or reverse walker. The presence of a strong, gentle horse worked magic on these children by allowing them a freedom of expression and movement they were unable to achieve for themselves when earthbound.

Winston Churchill has been famously quoted as saying, "There is something about the outside of a horse that is good for the inside of a man." I know this to be true in my own life, as the pleasures of horse ownership serve to both ground and inspire me. My horse gives me unconditional love, common sense, and wings to fly, and when I am with him I am unable to dwell upon negativity but am released to live in the moment. If a horse can do all that for me, a mere ordinary person, consider the possibilities for those less fortunate. Humans and horses have been inextricably linked together for more than four thousand years, with the horse providing transportation, food, and power for daily living and for war. With the modernization of the world and the industrial revolution, the horse's central role in family life waned but he was still recognized as a partner in sport and as a recreational platform for able-bodied and disabled riders alike. Classic hippotherapy has been around since the 1960s in America and Europe. The American Hippotherapy Association was formed in 1992, the year of my graduation from PT school.

The intention with hippotherapy is to have the horse's movement influence the rider, rather than the rider attempting to control the horse. Therapists direct the horse's movement in ways that stimulate responses in their patient's bodies that challenge posture, balance, strength, and mobility. There are striking parallels in the amount of body displacement that occurs when comparing the swing of the horse's back as he walks to the movement of the rider's pelvis, which facilitates motor control and ambulation ability in patients with movement dysfunctions. Horses can be made to walk faster or slower to give the patient more or less trunk motion, and can perform circles or lateral movements to enable weight shifting with shortening of a floppy side or lengthening of a collapsed or spastic side. Sitting backward on the horse promotes trunk extension, sitting astride stretches out tight hips and adductors, and lying prone across the horse's back can assist in elongating shortened spinal muscles. In essence, the horse becomes the ultimate interactive therapeutic modality.

All of these factors aside, the hippotherapy horse does so much more for the patient than simply promote function. Children with active minds who are forever trapped in the twisted wreckage of their bodies derive a huge psychological boost by suddenly being taller than all the surrounding adults. They become empowered by participating in a fun, social environment, and lose their hearts to "their" horse as they develop a special rapport.

During the five years that I worked part-time at the local hippotherapy center, I met so many bright young sparks. It was gratifying to see them initially come to the center shy and withdrawn, barely able to hold up their heads or sit unsupported, and then watch them graduate with greater independence and a full heart. Six-year-old Jake was one such child who arrived at the center in a wheelchair with a diagnosis of cerebral palsy and a seizure disorder. His vision was poor, and he required thick corrective lenses that were strapped onto his head so that when he involuntarily contorted into a full head, neck, and trunk extensor spasm, they would not fly off. His physician had approved of his participation with the "horse therapy," and his parents were eager for Jake to enjoy an outdoor experience that would simultaneously help him sit up taller so it would be easier for him to eat while giving him a break from his wheelchair. Mealtimes had long been a struggle for Jake, as his poor trunk control made it a supreme effort to hold his head up long enough to gain nutrition; Jake would become exhausted before being able to consume enough calories to grow.

At first, Jake seemed to be a serious child. Despite having no vocalization ability other than little squeaks and moans, he seemed able to understand everything we asked of him and tried his best to move until a wave of spasticity would rack his small body. We introduced him to Flash, his therapy horse, and waited to see if he would be afraid of this gentle chestnut giant. Instead of shrinking back, Jake smiled beatifically and reached out to gently bump Flash's nose with the back of his spastically clenched fist. They were instant friends.

Our treatments together were hard, yet fun, work. Initially Jake needed me to sit on Flash with him to help steady his frail body as Flash conscientiously plodded around the raked arena at the direction of our horse handler. Then, as Jake became stronger, I could walk alongside him while my partner and I each steadied one of Jake's legs on either side of Flash's narrow barrel, Jake himself supporting his upper body on a blue plastic therapy peanut. As time progressed, Jake's parents were thrilled with his progress and reported that not only were mealtimes much more successful but that Jake was finally beginning to gain weight and fill out his gaunt little frame. Every time Jake arrived at the center he would greet Flash with a squeal of delight and a huge smile that engulfed his thin face. In turn, Flash was especially careful to hold still so as not to knock the little boy over while Jake slowly patted Flash's soft, whiskery white nose.

When spring break arrived the horses had a week's rest while families all over the region went on vacation. When we returned to work the following week, we learned the sad news: Jake had been engulfed by a massive seizure from which he had inexplicably been unable to recover. Stricken, Jake's distraught parents left a heartbroken message on the clinic's answering machine to invite us to Jake's memorial service. When I heard the news I walked down to visit Flash and stroke his nose in Jake's honor, wondering how it was possible that such a vibrant little boy was no longer on the planet. At the memorial service there was Jake for one last time, the photograph depicting his huge grin as he pressed his cheek against Flash's broad, kind face.

It is not necessary for a child to be physically whole to be able to give and receive love. Jake and Flash had shared a special, loving connection with each other that left none of us untouched. After the memorial service, we all gathered together on the cemetery grounds to link hands and release yellow balloons into a sunlit blue sky and ponder grieving thoughts of loss over this very special child.

Part Two

The Spine

Our bodies are our gardens—our wills are our gardeners.
—William Shakespeare, English poet and playwright (1564–1616)

To "have a lot of backbone" means to have great strength of will and spirit. In this way, the spine is the figurative role model for the rest of the body. The spine literally provides the building blocks upon which we hinge our limbs to move and the means by which we are able to hold our heads up high. When injury occurs to this essential support column, quality of life can be grossly affected. The three natural curves of the spine include the cervical, thoracic, and lumbar sections, with the sacrum in place at the base of the spine to connect the spinal column to the bones of the pelvis. Some of us are blessed with straighter spines than others, but those who are decidedly curvier must make an extra effort to fight against the effects of gravity. My own backbone is quite prominent, with the spinous processes sticking out like the dorsal plates of a stegosaurus, and easily rounds as I lean over my patients. I have found that the constant need to correct my own posture in order to reduce personal muscle strain has turned out to be a blessing rather than a curse, as it gives me ample opportunity both to commiserate with my patients and also to implement my own treatment recommendations.

A Pain in the Neck

Would not love see returning penitence afar off, and fall on its neck and kiss it?
—*George Eliot, English novelist (1819–1880)*

The neck consists of seven cervical vertebrae (C1 through C7), which support the most important and delicate structures of the body. The carotid and vertebral arteries, jugular veins, lymph nodes, cervical nerve roots, and surrounding musculature are intimately arranged next to the spinal segments like pieces of a jigsaw puzzle. The cervical spine provides the essential link between our heads and our hearts, and is frequently the source of major discomfort. We can be "up to our necks in hot water" when in trouble or find another person a "pain in the neck" when they bother us. We "stick our necks out" when we take a risk, have someone "breathing down our neck" when we are being followed or threatened, are "hung from the neck until dead" if we commit a heinous crime, and can have a "millstone around our neck" when we feel that we are carrying a heavy burden.

~ ★ ~

Rita was a petite thirty-something woman with flashing, bright, birdlike eyes and dark, shoulder-length hair. She arrived at the clinic in search of relief from neck pain that had started after moving into the area from a faraway country. In the excitement of moving into her new home, Rita had "tweaked something" in her upper cervical spine. The first cervical vertebra, the atlas (C1), is named after the

Greek god Atlas, who is usually depicted as holding up the entire world on his shoulders. The atlas is the ring that connects the skull to the rest of the spine and allows us to politely nod our heads to each other. The atlas articulates with the second cervical vertebra, the axis (C2), which is the location at which approximately 50 percent of rotational movement occurs, allowing us to shake our heads in disagreement or to simply look to the side for oncoming traffic. Somehow in her dash among the moving boxes, or perhaps from being too agreeable (or otherwise!) with her husband, Rita had strained some of the small suboccipital muscles at the base of her skull that help control the movements of the atlas and the axis. Her symptoms included headaches, neck pain, and fatigue, all of which were interfering with the ability to decorate her new home and which made simple tasks such as driving unsafe.

Although this area of injury is frequently associated with poor posture or stress or anxiety, Rita exhibited all three. She chattered throughout the entire treatment session about how hard she was working on the house, how difficult it was for her to assimilate into her new neighborhood, how tough it was to help her twelve-year-old child with his homework, how little her husband was able to help her with anything at all due to his own full schedule, and how she felt powerless in the face of her pain. In her agitation, Rita continually raised her voice and talked over my responses, and as she described her life's troubles I could feel her chin jut forward and her suboccipital muscles clench into spasm as I attempted to work on loosening up her rigid neck.

"I cannot even drive now because the pain in my neck is so bad, I'm afraid to get behind the wheel! I can't turn my head or the pain just escalates. I can't use the computer or read a book for more than a few minutes because it triggers my pain, and even using the phone makes me scream. Well, it's one thing talking with a friend but when I'm on the phone for hours with the cable company to try to get the Internet working again, my neck just 'goes out' and I have to immediately take a pain pill and lie down. Then I asked my husband to do the simplest thing for me and he completely forgot, so I had to take care of it myself and then we had a big argument over it and it was a total crisis, and . . ."

"Rita, your neck muscles are—"

". . . he doesn't take me seriously! And then he promised to take me to the department store to buy some back-to-school items for my son but at the store we were fighting . . ."

"—getting tighter and tighter. This is what I mean by posture and stress adding to your symptoms. A lot of those things are out of your control, which is enhancing the cycle of pain and tension. Perhaps you could try pacing the activities that you know are going to be painful, for example—"

"... about whether we should buy him a blue or a black backpack. We simply could not agree ..."

"—when you know that using the computer or the telephone for longer than twenty minutes aggravates the feeling of tightness in your neck, why not try setting a timer and taking a small break after ten or fifteen minutes, before the pain builds. Then you can—"

"... and then my pain was too great and we had to leave the store. I was so angry, and then I tried folding some laundry but after ten shirts my neck was in agony. So, I took some pain pills and then I had a nap. When I woke up, I had to prepare the dinner but the chopping ..."

"Yes! So, you can practice this technique with the laundry too. Try folding only six shirts and then walk away before your pain starts, and go and do something else. Frequent changes of activity throughout the day will help you to—"

"... is unbearable. The position in which I must stand to use the knife raises my shoulder and my neck just shrieks and ..."

Pure adrenalin made my heart pound against my chest in response to Rita's incessant diatribe. No wonder her neck was constantly going into protective mode! I could feel my own neck tightening up as I vainly tried to defuse her anxiety. Finally, I was able to break through her discourse to show her a few postural strategies to help decrease the tension in her upper cervical muscles, and also asked her to consider keeping track of the type of activity and the duration of performing those activities that seemed to trigger her neck pain. Although I had no idea how else to help her, I felt that one way for her to break the cycle of pain and muscle tightness was to at least identify and then attempt to become empowered over her symptoms.

When I next saw Rita, she was rather quiet but seemed to be holding herself more comfortably. After exchanging pleasantries and assessing her neck range of motion and muscle tone, I could see and feel that her neck was a bit better. We reviewed some of her postural strategies ("lift your chest to face the sun, and slightly drop your chin so that your eyes remain level; but no military postures, please!"). Then, I began to gently mobilize the upper trapezius and suboccipital muscles that continued to display residual tightness.

As I worked with Rita, I debated whether to ask her how her life was going, but I was slightly fearful that I might inadvertently unleash another monologue on family disharmony. However, when Rita spoke, she remained calm and told me that she wanted to share her self-assessment with me. I told her that would be great, as in my patient care experiences, self-awareness was accurate much of the time.

She said, "I had quite a big crisis over the weekend, and it was very, very stressful, with a lot of family phone calls to and fro . . . despite this, I decided to reduce my pain medicine but found that after the crisis was over I actually had decreased neck pain and I felt that this depression or weight on me or whatever it was had lifted. I think that with me, there is a big connection between the mind and the body. Do you think this is a valid assessment?"

I breathed a sigh of relief. "I think you're right on. This tells me that you probably handled the crisis really well, and this success gave you confidence and helped you gain control over your life. This is an important lesson, because it gives you the opportunity to feel at less of a disadvantage in the midst of this transition period you're in."

"Yes, that's exactly it! I felt at a big disadvantage before, but now I feel better," she said.

"We handle ourselves differently when we're feeling stressed. If we had taken a picture of you last week when you were spinning around and feeling 'disadvantaged,' and then compared it to a picture taken today we would actually be able to measure a difference in the angles of your body and of the head on your neck," I said. "This could be a major factor for you, because keeping your neck in a more neutral position helps to keep the muscles that run from the shoulders to the neck and from the upper neck to the head much more relaxed, which decreases your pain."

"Is the psychological therapy part of the physical therapy in this country? You have so much psychological knowledge, but it must be very hard for you thinking all of the time!" Rita laughed.

"Actually, I had better be thinking of you while I work with you!" I responded. "But seriously, the patient is more than just the neck pain or the shoulder pain or whatever is going wrong. Each person is an individual with unique life circumstances that affect that pain. It just makes sense for me to try to acknowledge all of the factors that I can in my effort to help you and to speed up your healing process."

That day was a turning point for Rita. Once she started tuning in to her physical and her emotional habits, she was able to gain control over her symptoms, which in turn further improved her outlook and placed her on a positive spiral. This new pattern of self-awareness, postural correction, and pacing her stressful activities helped her lift the burden from her atlas and reduced the weight of the world on her shoulders.

As Rita became more confident, her demeanor changed such that she was less inwardly focused, becoming much more interested in others. One day as I was spotting her on a piece of exercise equipment, giving her feedback on keeping her shoulder blades down while performing the postural strengthening activity, I felt the intensity of her gaze on my face. Sure enough, she blurted out, "You are so fragile, so frail. I feel as if I could take a deep breath and blow you over!"

I laughed, "Let me refer you to a good ophthalmologist! Clearly, you're not able to see me properly from where you're standing."

"No, really! You seem so thin—if you were in my house, I would feed you up. What do you eat? Surely not more than a mere lettuce leaf a day. I hate lettuce, unless it is covered in chicken and mayonnaise."

This was a first, to be described in this way. I was of average size and build, and certainly in no danger of anorexia. Rita's observations must have been triggered by gazing at my thin cheeks. It's truly amazing how much you can get away with weight-wise if you have a thin face, although my face may be a bit more angular than some, since I do try to "choose my butt, not my face." The white lab coat can hide a lot of sins, but it was nice to know that the effects of my daily chocolate habit (the lure of my Dark Master, as my husband teases) were not obviously showing.

~ ★ ~

During the course of a career in physical therapy I have taken many continuing medical education (CME) courses to update my skills and practice new treatment techniques. Courses are offered all across the country by various experts renowned for their research, instruction, and thought-provoking approaches to patient care. Most CME courses have a limit on the number of attendees so that when the time comes to review or implement manual skills, therapists can easily practice on each other. Consequently, a colleague who actually suffers from a medical condition related to the topic in question creates an immediate, practical learning opportunity. Although the purpose of such courses is to become a better clinician, to refine palpation ability, and to build confidence, sometimes the experience goes astray.

I attended a cervical spine CME course on a fine November day that begged us to abandon the course and revel in the autumn sunshine. Nonetheless, we were all professionals and were content to focus on our task at hand: to review and palpate the upper cervical spinal anatomy. We paired up randomly and took turns lying prone on the provided treatment tables so that our partners could feel our necks. Since I have a long, skinny neck (swanlike, my husband insists), I am one of the easiest people in the world on whom to locate vertebral spinous and transverse processes, the places where muscles attach at their origins and insertions, and even the fronts of the vertebral bodies themselves. My partner, Barbara, however, was my polar opposite, with a short, thick neck and wrestler's physique. "Can't you feel how tight I am? My scalenes and upper trapezius muscles are like iron! And my suboccipitals—I defy you to find someone with a more tense neck," she exclaimed proudly as our instructor passed our table. Sighing, I stood back while he felt her upper neck at the base of the skull.

"Yes, you are rather tight here . . . class, gather 'round! Barbara has a trigger point in her obliquus capitis inferior—let's see if you can all locate that." My classmates all trooped over and lined up behind the preening Barbara, who was reveling in the attention. After twenty of us had gingerly felt her neck, the course instructor asked Barbara to turn over into a supine position.

"Now, I would like you all to perform manual traction on Barbara's neck to see how resistant this muscle can be when it's tight. One at a time, just get into the position—that's right—and apply a little distraction. No! Don't pull her head toward the ceiling, Donald, just a little cranial force, like you're trying to lift her head slightly away from her body and make her taller. Good, that's it. Next!"

And so we all lined up to pull on Barbara's neck. I was nearly the last to try, and by this time Barbara was looking less than thrilled by all the attention. I gently slipped my hands under her skull and lightly took hold . . .

"Arghh! What are you doing?" she screamed. "You have the worst hands I have ever felt in my life! It's like being mauled by a blacksmith! That's it, I've had enough, I'm outta here," she cried as she streaked off the table like a scalded cat and ran from the room.

Bewildered, I looked down at my fingers, my feelings hurt. Had I really touched her that callously? But I was known for my sensitive palpation skills in the clinic! As I puzzled over my apparent ineptitude, the instructor sidled up next to me. "Actually, this was nothing to do with you. She had just reached her saturation point. It happens." To this day I approach each new patient for the first time as if I am about to soothe a startled horse.

~ ★ ~

Pat turned toward the open door with a visible start as I knocked and entered, wishing him a good morning. "Hi honey, I sure hope you can help me out. I've been having the most terrible headaches, and I just can't seem to get to sleep at night. My doctor says it might be my neck acting up, but I don't know . . . she's ordering a brain MRI for me too, just to make sure I don't have a tumor. Do you think I might have a tumor? I'm so worried."

I murmured soothing noises to him as I took in the look on his face. Interestingly, he bore a strong resemblance to my mother's cousin but had an exhausted, pinched look about him that my relative fortunately lacked. I told him that I honestly had no idea about the tumor, but suggested that we look for other potential sources of his headache so that I might be able to help him while he waited for his MRI to get approved by his insurance. As I assessed his status, I found that his cervical range of motion was nearly normal except for the fact that he was almost completely unable to drop his chin toward his chest. Then, in response to my request, he looked up toward the ceiling.

"You know, honey, this makes me a little dizzy," Pat commented as he strained to lift his chin.

"Do you feel dizzy at other times?" I asked. "What about when you tilt your head back to shave? When you roll over in bed? Or when you're the passenger in a car?"

Pat looked a little gray, as if he was waiting for a wave of nausea to pass. "Yeah . . . I haven't been able to let my wife drive now for awhile. And come to think of it, sometimes it seems like if I get out of bed or turn my head too fast, I feel kinda dizzy too. It's really weird, like I've been drinking and the room is spinning around me."

I moved on to neurological tests. Pat's upper extremity sensation, muscle strength, and neural tension tests were all normal, although his deep tendon reflexes were bilaterally brisk. I asked him to lie down so I could palpate his neck. Pat took a long time to gingerly get into position on his stomach, and then had trouble relaxing his face down onto the towel. I gently began to feel the vertebral and muscular structures of his neck, and was astonished to find that he was almost completely rigid. "Pat, are you doing OK?" I asked with some concern. I felt a sudden wave of lightheadedness, and leaned against the treatment bench for support. Had I remembered to eat breakfast?

"Well, when you push there I feel a little dizzy again," he replied. I looked down at my thumbs and saw that I was carefully mobilizing one of the right upper cervical facet joints as he spoke. I tried the other side.

"How about this?" I enquired.

"Yeah, there too . . . and you know, I'm getting one of my headaches now," was the wondering reply.

That day I was able to reproduce most of Pat's symptoms by lightly pressing on the tight suboccipital muscles and underlying vertebrae. Our treatment program became very simple: Each time he came in for treatment, I would carefully help Pat to loosen up his tight cervical structures through gentle soft tissue and joint mobilization techniques, and then give him a home exercise program for some very basic vestibular stimulation exercises to help his inner ear adaptation. Pat seemed to be suffering from benign paroxysmal positional vertigo (BPPV), a condition in which position changes of the head and neck trigger a feeling of dizziness in response to the movement of tiny calcium carbonate crystals (otoconia) against the hair cells within the semicircular canals of the inner ear. He had become locked into a pattern of cervical guarding and tightness in response to his initial symptoms of dizziness; then, as his dizziness had worsened, triggered by very specific movements, he had unconsciously moved his neck less and less until he had become rigid. Of course, this relative immobility led to reduced input from the mechanoreceptors in his neck, further sensitizing his vestibular system. Ultimately, the muscular tightness had resulted in a series of tension headaches.

Several visits later, I was struck by how much Pat had regained his youth and vigor. Freed at last from most of the cervical tightness, headaches, and dizziness, his face looked like a bright, newly minted coin instead of a dingy gray sock. He was much more relaxed, and was no longer jumpy when I entered the room or if he heard a loud noise outside the door. Eventually, the long-awaited MRI turned out to be negative for tumors. Pat was able to embrace his life again, and I had no more instances of lightheadedness when treating him.

~ ★ ~

Magnetic resonance imaging (MRI) has become a fairly commonplace test, and in this country we are fortunate to have virtually immediate access to pictures of our internal systems whenever the need arises. Because MRI is ordered so frequently, I have tended to think of it almost as a glamorous cousin to the plain X-ray film— easily obtained, simple to do, but yielding wondrous results akin to viewing a picture through 3-D glasses. So after enduring many months of lower cervical stiffness, burning pain that radiated into my shoulder blade, and nonstop tingling in my left forearm and ring and little fingers, I finally decided to seek help.

Dr. R explored my neck range of motion (stiff), reflexes (brisk; I startle easi-ly), muscle strength (specific left arm weakness), sensation (intact), and neural tension (positive), and opted to send me for an MRI of my neck. Armed with his prescription for the test, I set off for the nearest imaging center and filled out the obligatory paperwork. When the staff questioned me about any tendencies I might have toward claustrophobia, I was able to truthfully answer that I had never had a problem. After being instructed to undress and leave all jewelry and personal items in the provided locker, I was led to the testing room. There stood the infamous tube. I was mildly curious about the procedure, having seen myriad test results from my patients and having heard their stories, but after all, I was a health professional myself, so this should be a piece of cake—there was nothing to fear.

I was asked to lie down on the hard, narrow ledge and told to stay as still as possible ("Try not to even swallow, dear"). The technician activated the ledge, and I began to slowly slide into the tube, head first. I confidently looked around, alertly taking in the process, when I saw the roof of the tube approach and then engulf my head. With the beige-colored ceiling inches from my nose, I could no longer see anything else. And then it happened. My heart exploded in my chest, banging to escape, and I could feel nothing but blind panic. It was like being buried alive inside a lighted coffin! Airless and cramped, I could feel my elbows lightly grazing the sides of the tube as I fought against my fear. No, I had to get out—"OK dear, we're going to start the first set. You'll hear some noises, but just try to lie still." Oh . . . I squeezed my eyes shut, heart racing and adrenalin surg-ing. I frantically talked to myself, trying to reason that I knew where I was, that I could push the panic button anytime and leave, that it was a simple MRI test that thousands of people went through every day . . . I was panting in short, ragged gasps, trying to stay as motionless as possible and determined not to give in to my terror.

One more minute, I can lie here for just one more minute . . . I visualized standing outside in a grassy, sunlit field. Then I imagined I was grooming my horse, carefully picking out his feet before going riding along a ridge with a sweeping view of the Pacific Ocean. For forty-five long minutes I played mental games with myself as my heart hammered in my chest and threatened to burst out through my throat, my panic unabated. Finally, I was rewarded with the moving hum of the ledge sliding me back out from the casket of death. I was free—and could barely stand up after my emotional workout. Never again would I take lightly my patients who suffer anxiety.

The MRI results came in, showing a fair amount of wear and tear. A few sloppy bulging discs here, some bone spurs there, and a retrolisthesis, or area where one of my vertebrae had slipped backward on the one below, probably from repeatedly looking down at my patients as I treated them. All of it was ammunition to work on my posture more effectively to help keep my nerve roots from becoming pinched as I worked.

The aftereffects of that day stayed with me for a long time. For weeks I had to drive my car with the windows rolled down, treat my patients with the door ajar, and keep away from movie theaters and other enclosed spaces. For months when I visited the bookstore I could only examine the new releases that were displayed on tables near the front door, because if I tried to move further into the building I would feel the panic rising in my throat again. Over time I was able to slowly desensitize myself, but I continue to feel a whole new respect for the primal "fight or flight" urge that lasts to this day.

~ ★ ~

I have always loved hot weather, having been continually deprived of comforting heat throughout my childhood. My parents' internal thermostats had always kept them toasty warm, and their idea of bundling up was to nudge the windows closed against the damp, foggy gloom of San Francisco and put on a light poly-ester cardigan or long-sleeved shirt. However, I finally discovered that it's possible to have too much of a good thing. One summer my husband I were driven to sleep downstairs on our hunt-scene tapestry sofa bed to avoid becoming inciner-ated in our west-facing bedroom upstairs, and here I discovered true neck pain for the first time. My neck had been fussy for a long time because of the need to continually look down at my patients on the treatment tables and the occasionally awkward positions I would contort myself into to deliver a mobilizing force, but it had always returned to normal after a relatively short refractory period. However, one night on the dreaded tapestry sofa was my undoing.

After a hot, restless night, I woke before the alarm went off to the sound of a soft moaning noise. Startled, I attempted to raise my head from my pillow to dis-cover three things: one, my pillow had disappeared into the great divide between the back of the sofa and the mattress; two, I was completely unable to lift, move, or turn my head due to a dagger apparently stuck in the base of my neck; and three, I was the one making the noises, not some wild, wounded animal who had mistakenly wandered into our living room. It actually hurt to breathe.

Somehow, during the great pillow migration I had slept peacefully undisturbed with my neck in a position of combined extension, side bending, and rotation that slammed the right lower cervical facet joints together at the cervicothoracic junction. With a full patient list ahead of me I had to unstick myself—and fast. Engaging my husband's help, I was able to slide my head off the bed along with the rest of me and head for the shower with a nonsteroidal anti-inflammatory cocktail in my hand. After warming up the muscle spasms and carefully readjusting the car mirrors so that I could see to drive without actually moving my neck, I headed off to work. Each bump in the road was agony and each intersection an ocular workout as I carefully scanned for cross traffic without turning my head, but I managed to pull into the underground garage without scraping the metallic charcoal-gray paint off my fenders. The first person on my list was, of course, a neck patient.

Michael was normally seen by my colleague, so this was to be our first meeting. As I gingerly climbed the clinic stairs at 7:20 a.m., I found a thirty-five-year-old sandy-haired man slumped pathetically on the low retaining wall of the atrium fountain. "Well, it's about time," he commented as I stiffly strode up to the office door, keys in hand. I glanced at him out of the corner of my eye, feeling my eyebrows indignantly disappear under my hair. Swallowing my irritation, I replied, "You must be Michael—pleased to meet you! Although it sounds like we have our wires crossed. The clinic doesn't actually open for another ten minutes, you know."

He said nothing in response, but straightened up to follow me into the clinic. "Please relax for a moment while I put my stuff down, and then we can get started right away," I offered. Michael audibly sighed in a begrudging manner, but sat sullenly in the reception area while I bustled about flipping on the lights and rotating the Levolors into an open position. The two messages flashing on the overnight answering machine would just have to wait.

"Come on back," I invited as I delicately eased on my lab coat, trying not to move my neck, and picked up his chart. "Jack filled me in on your case already," I said. "You had originally hurt your neck at the C6/C7 vertebral level last year in a work-related motor vehicle accident, is that right? How are things feeling right now? Jack said that the last time he saw you a few weeks ago, things were going well for you and your workers' compensation adjustor was talking about wrapping up your case."

"Yeah, things were really good until I went skiing over the holidays and took a fall . . . but I did OK until I got home again a few days ago. Since then I've had really strong pain in my neck."

"Is this in the same area of your neck as before or a different location?"

"This time, it's in my left shoulder blade area."

"On a scale of zero to ten, zero being no pain at all and ten being the worst pain you can imagine, a level that would make you go directly to the hospital, what is your pain level?"

"Right now it's about a two out of ten." Arghh. With my own neck feeling like it had an ice pick sticking out of it, a solid pain level of seven despite the anti-inflammatories, I had to summon my inner Mother Teresa.

"I see . . . so at rest you feel fairly good. Are there any positions or activities that increase your pain, and if so, how strong does the pain get at its worst?"

"At its worst, my neck can be a five or a six. It feels pretty good most of the time, but stress and work really get it going. Sometimes, when it's bad like that I have to take a Darvocet. I mean, the weekends and stuff are OK and I can play a round of golf without any trouble, but by the end of the workday it can be pretty bad."

"All right then; let's take a look at you."

I wasn't able to demonstrate neck movement for him as I usually did with patients without squeaking in pain, so instead I simply asked Michael to put his neck through its normal range of motion, first looking down with his chin toward his chest, then lifting his chin to look up at the ceiling. Then, I directed him to tilt his head into right and then left cervical side bending, followed by turning his head each direction for cervical rotation. None of the movements appeared restricted, and Michael reported no pain with movement. I quickly rechecked his upper extremity deep tendon reflexes and muscle strength—no deficits there. Tests of upper limb neural tension, in which the arms are individually slowly moved into positions that take up the slack of the major nerve tracts, were also negative. Finally, I requested that Michael lie prone on the treatment table so that I could palpate his cervical and upper thoracic areas.

Careful vertebral mobilization, in which the therapist specifically presses upon the spinous and transverse processes of each vertebra, revealed no segmental stiffness or pain. With my own neck burning at the right cervicothoracic junction and shoulder blade as I stiffly looked down at Michael's neck, I began to cautiously assess his muscle tone. Everything felt normal. Were my palpation skills on the fritz, my ability to sense masked by my own neck pain? OK, focus: Suboccipital muscles—check. Cervical paraspinals—check. Upper and middle trapezius—check. Rhomboids—check. Levator scapulae—mildly hypertonic at the left scapular border. Michael groaned, "Ah, that's it! It's killing me!"

"Michael, are you left-handed by any chance?"

"Yeah, as a matter of fact, I am. Why?"

"Do you use the computer mouse with your left hand? Hold the phone in your left hand? Do you use a thin old pillow, or have you woken up in an awkward position recently?"

"Yeah—actually, I fell asleep in my chair in front of the TV a few days ago and woke up with this pain."

The levator scapulae muscle is generally innervated by the third and fourth cervical nerve roots with some additional innervation by the dorsal scapular nerve of C5; however, nerve pathways can be highly individualized in different people, somewhat like the wandering tributaries of a river. The levator muscle itself originates at the transverse processes of the first four cervical vertebrae and inserts into the inner corner of the scapula, and it was here that I could feel a little increased muscle tone in Michael's upper back. Since the muscle typically acts to raise the shoulder blade, falling asleep with the head hanging in a position of tension might have overstretched the muscle and then caused it to retract in spasm.

I hazarded a guess. "I think that this probably has little to do with stress or work, but after you strained it the other day your terrible posture makes it worse as the day goes on! Listen, Michael, I think that your problem might be solved if you straighten up your posture throughout the day and quit sleeping in your recliner." In solidarity, I made a mental note never to sleep on my own sofa again.

Michael absorbed my scolding with good grace and recognized that my theory might at least in part be right. He became quite friendly, telling me all about his skiing trip, his job, his wife, and his dream of becoming a massage therapist. Deep tissue mobilization of his trigger point at the levator scapulae combined with a promise to change his postural habits dealt with Michael's pain, and later in the day my colleague relieved me of my own right C6/7 facet pain with a short session of specific segmental spinal mobilization.

Mimicking Quasimodo

The best way to knock the chip off your neighbor's shoulder is to pat him on the back.
—*Author unknown*

The thoracic spine consists of twelve closely stacked vertebrae that surround the spinal cord and serve as a sturdy tent pole from which the ribs are suspended. The ribs themselves provide a protective cage around the all-important heart and lungs, and in conjunction with the thoracic spine act as a platform for upper extremity muscle attachments that enable us to reach, hug, and lift up our children and pets for affection.

Nowhere else in the body can we find an area so easily influenced by the effects of gravity and our mental attitudes. We slump when we are tired, hunch down in an effort to minimize ourselves when we feel self-conscious, "square our shoulders" by lifting our sternums and extending our thoracic spines when we feel confident or aggressive, and flex our thoracic spines into a fetal position when we feel vulnerable or depressed. The transitional area between the end of the thoracic spine and beginning of the lumbar spine is the region where the naturally forward, kyphotic, curve of our thoracic spine must literally change direction and blend into the naturally arched, lordotic curve of the lumbar spine. Sometimes, this transitional area creates problems for us when we are actually in the midst of a pivotal transition period in life.

~ ★ ~

I have always known a deep-seated love of horses, despite a relatively horse-free childhood growing up in the chilly, crowded hills of San Francisco. Frequent visits to our English family enabled me to spend the summers hanging out at the local stables mucking out stalls, cleaning tack, and brushing ponies to earn an occasional soul-stretching ride. Many years later when I completed my undergraduate education, one of my classmates gave me her majestic gray horse, "because I know you'll give him a great home for the rest of his life." Prophetic words, indeed. Euphoric, I cared for and loved William throughout many happy years of competition and a well-earned retirement until the end of his days. My second great horse, Riley, also came to me unexpectedly. Injured and quirky, the bay Irish thoroughbred had been abandoned in a small pen with no one to care for him until I learned of his plight. We immediately clicked with each other as kindred spirits, and no one rode him but me—until I met my husband.

As Jim and I steadily discovered more about each other throughout the dating process, my then-future husband could see that the horses in my life were a permanent fixture; so, he decided to join me on my rides rather than rail against his newfound fate. On one cloudy winter's day we went out to see the horses together and decided to work on our form in the neighbor's arena. Jim vaulted easily onto Riley, and after a brief warm-up began to practice a few transitions between trot and canter. Then, Riley appeared to have a flashback to unhappier times. No doubt startled by something that Jim and I could not hear and then fearing punishment, Riley decided to flee to safety and took off as fast as he could, rapidly becoming unstoppable in his panic. Time instantly warped into fast-forward, and my husband-to-be was suddenly unhorsed and awkwardly lying on the ground on his back, winded and in tremendous pain. "Don't move!" I cried, racing to his side. Grimly, Jim gritted his teeth and, muttering "a good horseman always gets right back on," stiffly remounted a chastened Riley. A brief circuit later, and, with honor satisfied, we pushed Riley into his paddock and set off for the hospital. In the emergency room we were enlightened as to the cause of Jim's tremendous pain—he had sustained a wedge compression fracture of the T12 vertebra. It was then I discovered that my future husband was a true warrior with a tremendously high pain tolerance as he battled the intense muscle spasms that assaulted him throughout his recovery without medication. Thankfully, Jim's life transition experience of dating me wasn't enough to put him off for good, and he eventually forgave Riley and decided to marry me anyway.

~ ★ ~

"Sorry I'm late! I decided to take my bath last night instead of in the morning to save time, but then discovered that I still needed to wash my face, comb my hair, massage lotion into my feet, and struggle to get my support hose on."

I encouraged Edith to follow me into one of the treatment rooms with a smile, and settled her onto a table lying on her left side. "So, you decided to 'go Victorian' with your bathing habits?" I enquired. Edith smiled questioningly at me, encouraging me to continue.

"Well, in Victorian times those hardworking maids would wake up each day in total darkness and spring out of bed in their shifts, where they would have to first break the ice on the surface of their water ewers before being able to use the freezing water to wash with. Then, they would quickly grab a flannel and wash their faces, armpits, and between their legs (in that order) before hurriedly donning their uniforms and racing downstairs to begin sweeping out the grates and lighting the fires for the day."

Edith smiled wider and said that since she would have been the mistress of the house and not the servant, she would have asked her parlor maid to bring the hip bath into her room so that she could wash in warm comfort before the fire prior to getting dressed. As we pursued this flight of fancy, I worked on Edith's back. Her thoracic spine was twisted sideways in a Quasimodo hump of scoliosis, and was also excessively kyphotic due to her underlying osteoporosis and generally collapsing spine. Edith's head crested my lower sternum when we stood side by side in front of the treatment mirror to work on her posture. She had always been petite, but after a series of spontaneous compression fractures and her natural tendency to hunch forward, bowed by gravity's invisible pull, she was now diminutive and frail. The strength of her mind belied her appearance, and we had many bright conversations about the state of the world, human nature, and what to wear as we worked together.

"Ah, that's a bad spot," Edith flinched, as I gently pressed on a muscle spasm nestled against her midthoracic spine. The spasm was at the convexity of her scoliotic curve and was a frequent source of pain due to the constant stretching pull of her thoracic paraspinal muscles as they struggled against the inexorable lean of her spine. Her other problem area was in the opposite thoracolumbar paraspinal group, on the left side, where her curve was most concave. In this spot, the muscles would be forever shortened as her spine slowly collapsed toward her hip.

Scoliosis is a difficult problem to treat, especially in the elderly, as it insidiously continues to worsen over time. Edith was caught in a vice of her body's own making, which was now rapidly accelerating its pressure as her very bones crumbled inside her. So far, she had derived great relief from physical therapy treatment as we explored a combination of gentle deep tissue mobilization to reduce her spasms, breathing exercises to open her folding ribcage, and postural strengthening exercises to help her battle gravity's relentless force. She sighed in appreciation as I carefully released her spasms, her watery blue eyes magnified into pools of light behind her thick glasses, saying, "This is so much more helpful than that other therapy place. All they did was talk to me for five minutes then show me some exercises to do in the gym by myself! I was never sure if I was doing them right, and I never felt any improvement."

After gently ironing the kinks out of her bent form as best I could, I began reviewing breathing and posture. I asked, "Now, Edith, are you lifting your chest up one thousand times a day? Anywhere you happen to be, you can do this. When you hear the phone ring, lift your chest. When you're driving and stop at a light, lift your chest. When you're watching a program on TV, lift your chest at the beginning of each commercial and again at the end. Each time you 'fix' yourself, you're reminding your spine to straighten up a bit, which lets your muscles relax for a moment. Then, by the end of the day, your pain won't have built up so much."

"You have an answer for everything," she laughed. "Now, what can I do about this?" she asked jokingly, pulling her frayed bra strap out from under her shirt. "I simply cannot find a good front-closing bra that isn't in a racer-back style! It's the only kind I can wear since I can't reach behind my back by myself around that hump, and I hate to keep asking my husband to help me—he says he'd rather help me get undressed."

I laughed. "I know just what you mean—and you know, I have the same exact problem. I can reach behind my back but my spine is so bony I can't stand the pressure of those hooks digging into me, especially when I sit down and lean against the back of a chair."

Commiserations aside and one detailed Internet search later, I solved our shared problem. Certain aspects of thoracic spine comfort can be found in front-closing bliss.

~ ★ ~

While my English mother was sent to boarding school to keep her safe from falling bombs, my American father fled to California to escape the relative deprivation of his own childhood and pursue his dreams. As a result, my parents concocted a plan for my brother and me that would remove us from rationing and despair. We were adequately fed, and were both destined to go to college and create better lives for ourselves than my parents had known in their youth. According to plan, we cleaned our plates and applied ourselves to our studies; but, in my efforts to keep up with my six-foot-four-inch brother, I overate myself into chunkiness by the age of thirteen. Until I regained control over my appetite, I compensated by rounding my upper back and shoulders in a futile attempt to minimize the extra pounds on my five-foot-eight-inch frame. By the age of sixteen I had graduated from high school, shed my teenage angst, and trimmed the fat, but my hunching habit worsened as I dwelled in my deep-seated desire not to draw attention to myself.

Part of the enjoyment of PT school lies in discovery, not just about kinesiology, anatomy, physiology, and motor learning, but also about how the particular body you have been blessed with stacks up against the norm. As we learned about normal and abnormal anatomy in our lab sessions, our instructors would select one or another of us to demonstrate some characteristic as an example for the rest of the class. This privilege was nervously anticipated, because although we secretly hoped that we were special in some way, we also feared being held up as an example of some bizarre, previously unknown, condition. My turn to be "demo" arrived when we were learning about the thoracic spine. First, my classmate Jessica was invited to the front of the room. The instructor had her turn sideways so that she could exhibit her profile to the class, and she then molded a bendable art ruler along Jessica's back. Straight as an arrow, very nice. Then, I was invited up. I obediently turned sideways alongside Jessica and stood erect with the Queen's posture, feeling the pressure of a second ruler being applied against my back. I had always been quite flexible, so felt confident that my regal pose would be recorded in flattering detail. As the ruler left my back, I turned with a smile . . . and was shocked to see how dreadfully bent into kyphosis my spine truly was. "You can see that Jessica's Asian heritage has helped to give her a lovely straight spine, as compared to Anne's," my instructor informed the class. I went to sit down with tears blinding my eyes, unable to hear another word. How deformed I was! And I had actually been trying to stand up straight for once.

After class, the instructor came up to me. "I could see you were upset in there about how the shape of your spine looked on the ruler. Everyone's different—not good or bad. It's actually a benefit to you that you have this awareness at a young age, because now you can do something about it! Spend some time each day working on your posture, and don't let gravity take advantage of you. Plus, this will give you great sympathy for your future patients. There are no people out there with perfect bodies."

~ ★ ~

Lily flicked aside the royal blue patient gown, exclaiming, "My pain is here . . . and here . . . and here" as she gestured at the curve of her bare ribcage. Averting my eyes from her left breast, I squinted warily at her side. The ribs appeared normal, but as they wrapped around her body from front to back they were cruelly divided by a livid red scar that ended at her spine. Lily was in physical therapy for treatment of debilitating chest wall pain following cancer surgery, and had requested a female therapist to help her with her treatment. The surgery had involved a long incision and retraction of her ribs to allow the thoracic surgeon unfettered access to her lungs. Lily did not have lung cancer but was suffering from colon cancer that had metastasized into the pulmonary tissues. As I looked at her deep scar, I wondered. The metastatic process always seems incredibly sinister to me—how do cancer cells, recognizable under a microscope by their own particular size and shape, break free and swim relentlessly through the tributaries of the body's blood and lymphatic vessels before deciding to take up residence in a different part of the body? Do the cells get restless in their never-ending quest for body domination? Why does this always seem to happen to the nicest people?

The only other time I had seen a patient with such pervasive scars was after my mother-in-law's thoracotomy the previous year. She too had been diagnosed with cancer, although in her case it had originated close to the lungs in the lower esophagus. Her incisional pain was constant, and produced sweeping muscle spasms along the side of her chest. Unfortunately, my attempts to alleviate her pain had been completely ineffective, and her spasms were triggered over and over again as she struggled not to cough up blood.

Lily's eyes teared as she stood before me, her face mutely appealing to me for help. "I can't sleep, and the pain . . . it's all over my back, and chest, and breast. I can't even walk without holding my ribs, because it feels like my ribs are folding together." I examined her thoracic spine range of motion and found that she was unable to bend forward without stabbing anterior chest pain, yet was unable to stretch backward into full extension due to a pinching pain where her ribs met her spine. Her left arm was clamped protectively against her side, and any attempt to raise the arm produced a burning pain in her axilla. Palpation revealed severe spasms in the left intercostals, latissimus dorsi, pectorals, rotator cuff, trapezius, and thoracic paraspinals. I smiled at her encouragingly as she winced beneath my gentle touch, saying, "Well, we can certainly identify the areas of tightness! I won't have any problem honing in on which muscles need work."

I began with the lightest form of myofascial release imaginable, propping Lily up in a sitting position leaning onto a pile of pillows since she could not lie down comfortably on the firm treatment table. I sat next to her on a rolling stool, using cupped hands and wide fingers to carefully deliver pressure to her tender side. She was a silent sufferer, only letting me know if I hovered too long over one spot by quietly holding her breath. Neither of us spoke. I allowed my healing fingers to be guided by her taut muscles, and was rewarded by a gradual release of tension as I worked. Suddenly, she let out a long sigh and straightened up. "Better." In unspoken harmony, we moved her onto her right side to lie on a nest of pillows on the treatment table. Here I could finally move her left arm through its natural range of motion, releasing it away from its constant job of guarding her left side. By the end of the session, Lily could walk short distances without holding her ribcage and had lost her strained expression.

Over subsequent visits, Lily improved steadily. Her muscles slowly released one by one, and she reported being able to lift her small grandson again. As she healed, so did I. Although my mother-in-law had already passed on, it was as if I could finally release some of her pain and restore a thread of bodily harmony through Lily, despite not being able to directly help her during our time together in this life.

~ ★ ~

Each person craves respectful treatment by others, especially when the area of injury is in a more "personal" region. Treatment of disorders relating to the thoracic area can involve much more than just the spine itself. Sometimes this is a major cause of embarrassment, especially when rib or pectoral muscle disorders necessitate treatment near the breast. Although I am comfortable with all types of anatomy, I have always taken great care to adequately drape my patients with towels and gowns so they can relax and feel at ease while I work on them. One day I had an experience that made me even more aware of the importance of respecting someone's personal privacy.

I had already put off going to the Willow Pavilion for my mammogram for four months. I kept trying to justify the delay to myself by thinking, "If I wait another few months, the scan will be late enough to apply to next year!" But in my case, breast self-examination was futile, like trying to feel for a rare agate inside a sock filled with rocks. I finally forced myself to at least book the appointment, secure in the knowledge that if I phoned that day, the likelihood of actually finding an opening before the following year was nearly impossible. But my head was abruptly pulled from the sand—the helpful voice on the other end of the telephone assured me they had an opening in the mammography schedule that very afternoon, if I wished to come in after lunch. I did not wish, but with a sigh made the appointment anyway, feeling that I was being prodded by fate.

After lunch I quickly went through the ritual of washing under my arms, to remove all traces of deodorant, and put on a clean shirt. Once at the Pavilion, I scanned the familiar form, checking off the same boxes as I did each year (why couldn't they just refer to my records? I could never remember how long it had been since my latest biopsy). Finally, I was ushered into the waiting area, where I removed the clothing from my upper body while examining the nipple markers on the pad attached to the changing room wall left behind by scores of other women. Why did some women leave their markers in the center of the panel and others in the border region? Was this a hidden camera self-esteem test of some kind? One marker was placed all alone on the upper left corner—where was its mate? Had its owner suffered a mastectomy, and only had one remaining breast left to mark? Why was the waiting area always suffused with tension and fear, even though most of us were there only to have a routine mammogram? My reverie was interrupted by the technician, who was bright and brisk.

She showed me into the X-ray cubicle, confirmed that I knew all about the need for compression, and then said, "OK, drop your robe," as she busied herself with the X-ray plates. I stood dumbly, thinking I had misheard. She repeated her request, and gazed at me expectantly while I slowly complied. Never in all my years in and around the medical profession had anyone ever asked me to simply strip down in front of them. I always took special care with my own patients to make sure they felt covered and safe. Even when apparently unself-conscious patients began to undress in front of me, I would leave the room or at least turn my back. Feeling horribly exposed, I stood as the technician strapped on the lead apron and led me over to the X-ray machine, proceeding to manipulate my breasts, arms, and hips into position. I stared straight ahead, thinking that it must just be faster for her to not bother attempting to keep me, the patient, warm and draped. Four views later on each side it was over.

The technician opened the door, clutching my films in her hands, before I had the change to regain my robe. People were passing in the corridor outside, conversing and curiously glancing into my cubicle. "Just wait here in case we need to take an extra shot," she said, "I'll be right back." I sat down with humiliated resignation, clutching my robe loosely about me without bothering to tie it, as I had never yet escaped without the frightening "extra views." Not only were my breasts extremely fibrocystic and dense, but I had already endured six biopsies that had left me with generous amounts of scar tissue. My plight had turned into a standing joke with my general surgeon, and every time I left him I would say, "See you in another year or two!" So far I had been lucky, and everything had turned out to be benign.

As predicted, the technician returned with another chirpy, "Just flip off your robe again for me!" before completing the extra views. As I stood there exposed in my goose-pimpled upper body nakedness, I vowed to renew my vigilance over my own patients' privacy rather than make them parade in front of me like a prize heifer at the county fair.

The Cost of Walking Upright

And yet not turn your back upon the world.
—*Henry Wadsworth Longfellow, American poet (1807–1882)*

The lumbar spine is constructed from five thick, dense vertebrae that provide the link between the pelvis and the rest of the trunk and neck. This region is what sets us apart from the animal kingdom and enables us to walk upright and to make love face-to-face. However, the lumbar spine can also be a source of great pain; despite the fact that we spend up to one-third of our lives resting in bed, low back pain is one of the most common reasons for missed work. It is thought that up to 80 percent of us will experience some sort of low back pain during at least one point in our lives as the result of trauma, degenerative changes, poor body mechanics, or sloppy posture.

~ ★ ~

Sandra was already lying on her back on the treatment table when I entered the room. At first glance, the slender, dark-haired twenty-nine-year-old seemed to be at a low risk for chronic back pain. She looked athletic and fit, and younger than the age penned lightly onto the patient questionnaire. As I introduced myself, Sandra lifted her slight form up and sprawled awkwardly with one leg on each side of the treatment table, extending her hand for me to shake. Here I found my first clue—she was a "motor moron," with the body control of a poorly manipulated puppet. Her hand grazed mine and flopped to her side as she reached out, swinging her legs jerkily over the edge of the table and narrowly missing her huge tan leather briefcase with her right foot. Inside the briefcase I could see a sheaf of untidy papers, a small bottle of water, and a huge bag of potato chips.

Our introductions made, I began to ask her about her condition. Throughout our interview she remained standing, her weight shifting from leg to leg as she continually fidgeted like a leggy young colt. While she stood, she "hung on her ligaments," a therapy term to describe patients who stand without any engagement of the trunk muscles. In this position, patients will hyperextend their knees and lumbar spine, thrusting their hips and pelvis forward as they balance against gravity in an exaggerated model's stance. In Sandra, the posture was accentuated by an enormous belt pack, upon which her cell phone was strung along the front of her stomach.

Sandra told me that she was no longer able to work because she could not sit down for longer than thirty minutes at her computer, but went for walks in the mornings and evenings and was able to play soccer with her small six-year-old son. Then, realizing her mistake, she clammed up. Since she was a workers' compensation patient, it wasn't terribly wise of her to fill me in on the details of her extracurricular activities. Consequently, it took me a long time to extract any additional information from her about previous injuries, her general state of health, and any medications she might be taking for her back. As I methodically went through the parameters of a lumbar evaluation, I found that her ailment was incredibly hard to pinpoint. Sandra performed her lumbar range of motion tests like a deflating balloon, collapsing forward without warning to touch the toes of her filthy white tennis shoes and then flopping backward into extension like a broken doll. Her reflexes were so brisk and erratic that I had to duck to avoid getting kicked in the head as I knelt before her patellar tendons with my rubber-tipped hammer. She said that she had normal sensation but often felt "fuzzy" in the legs at random times of the day. When I asked her to lie on her stomach so that I could see her back, she flopped violently onto her back, face up.

"Thanks, but I want to see your back, not have you lie on your back," I gently encouraged.

After a brief tussle, she removed her massive belt pack and got comfortable on her stomach so that I could look at and feel her back. As I slightly lifted her shirt, I was confronted with two large X's freshly marked on her back with black felt-tip pen.

"It looks like you've had an epidural injection or two recently," I commented.
"Yes," she laconically replied.

I asked, "How long ago did that happen?"

"About ten days ago," she said.

I inwardly recoiled—it looked like Sandra hadn't bothered to bathe in ten whole days. When I first assess a spine, I usually observe the area for anomalies in the shape and appearance of the back, and then gently press on the spinous and transverse processes to test each vertebral level for stiffness and pain. I continue the information-gathering process by putting some lotion on my hands and then palpating the muscles and soft tissues along the spine, sacrum, and hips. (Using lotion enables me to feel the deeper tissues rather than become distracted by the friction of the dermal layer). But as I gently applied my fingertips to Sandra's back, the lotion under my hands turned gray and then black with dirt. Shuddering, I averted my eyes from the growing mud pie and tried to concentrate on what I was feeling. Muscle spasms typically feel like dense, thickened wads of tissue beneath the fingers, but underneath Sandra's greasy filth lurked thin, flat muscles that felt as if they hadn't been activated in years. Her weary thoracolumbar paraspinals felt too atrophied to be able contract, let alone go into spasm. Years of poor body mechanics, sloppy habits, and terrible posture had conspired with severe trunk weakness and innate hypermobility to cause her back pain. When she stood up, she drooped into end range extension and ground the bones and cartilage of her facet joints together, narrowing the sensitive spaces around her spinal nerves. When she sat, she slumped into end range flexion and placed tremendous force upon her beleaguered discs. The only solution was exercise to awaken Sandra's somnolent muscles into protecting her bruised and battered infrastructure, and education to improve and coordinate her way of moving.

It has been said that it takes at least one hundred days to break an old habit and replace it with a new one. Sandra and I had our work cut out for us, and in the multiple days ahead we struggled to coordinate her gangling limbs into positions that allowed her overwhelmed spine some relief. Every exercise was fraught with peril as Sandra allowed her spine to snap back and forth between end range flexion and extension despite my pleas to control the excessive movement using her core abdominal muscles. I felt as if I was on an endless loop as I struggled to convince Sandra of the importance of controlling her unruly body. Slowly, we began to make headway. Sandra's trunk muscles finally began to assume a more active role, and I was no longer able to nearly push her over with a tiny pressure of my finger. The potato chips in the briefcase remained a constant, but Sandra herself started to shape up and embrace a smoother way of moving as her pain levels decreased.

~ ★ ~

I winced as the spine specialist flicked on the light box where it hung suspended on the wall. The X-rays were illuminated from behind with stark clarity, showing mostly bone with very little space where the discs and nerves would ordinarily reside. I glanced at my mother, who was seated beside me, waiting trustingly for the surgeon's verdict. She had been having difficulty walking for a long time, and I had suspected that lumbar spinal stenosis was at the center of her pain. My mother was of stoic North Yorkshire stock and never complained about anything physical, but I had noticed how frequently she needed to sit and rest on our outings. It had gotten to the point that wherever we went, she immediately scanned the room for a chair before she was able to relax, becoming panicky if there was none available. Once sitting, her back pain and stiffness would rapidly go away, but getting back up out of the desired chair was sometimes difficult. "My legs feel tired and weak," she would say. I finally confronted her, and she admitted that she was only really comfortable when lying on her right side in bed; even then, when she tried to turn over, she felt as if she were a stale bread roll being torn in half. We had talked about therapy-related exercises that might open up her spinal spaces and free her nerves from compression, but things were steadily worsening.

The X-rays were the worst I had ever seen. There were multilevel thoracic compression fractures, razor-sharp protruding points on each lumbar vertebra, and giant spearlike bone spurs projecting from numerous locations all over the thoracolumbar spine. The biggest calcified whale tooth was sticking out on the right side, near the place my mother would point to as the ripping bread roll area. "You have DISH," proclaimed the surgeon. "Also known as diffuse idiopathic skeletal hyperostosis, or Forestier's disease, DISH manifests as back pain and stiffness." He pointed to the posterior vertebral bodies in the lateral X-ray view. "Here you can see how the posterior longitudinal ligament has already turned into bone . . ." the surgeon indicated the right side of the anterior-posterior (AP) view, ". . . and here you can see the classic right-sided osteophyte formation across many levels of the spine."

My mother shifted in her seat, turning to me for an explanation. "But, what does it mean?" she asked.

"Well look at all the bone spurs; some of those are rubbing against the nerves in your back," I said. Turning to Dr. T, I asked, "It all looks pretty tight in there. Can anything be done to open up some of those spaces?"

He replied, "The good news is she doesn't need surgery. There just isn't much I can do in there, other than surgically decompress and then fuse the spine." He smiled at my Mom, "But, if you wait a little longer, your back will fuse itself; it's already trying! The bad news is that if you've already tried physical therapy, there isn't anything I can offer you other than a spinal epidural injection to help control the pain."

I asked, "But there seem to be two kinds of pain—the right-sided pain she feels when she's turning over in bed, and the low back pain and leg weakness she feels when she tries to stand and walk for any distance." My mother nodded in agreement.

Dr. T concurred as he pointed toward the narrowed spaces where the spinal nerves normally exited the spine. "There is such a lot of extra bone here that the spine has a difficult time moving anywhere without pain. The DISH itself is probably causing the turning-in-bed pain, and the spinal foraminal stenosis is causing the mobility pain. I would suggest that you do an MRI . . ." his voice trailed off as my mother began to vigorously shake her head.

"There's no way I can have an MRI. I'd just freak out in there!" she exclaimed fearfully.

"It would be the only way to see if you have central canal stenosis, which might explain your standing and walking pain," he cajoled.

I interrupted, "But if there's nothing we can do for it, there's not much point putting her through that." Apparently my mother was wildly claustrophobic—had I inherited the tendency from her? After more discussion about treatment alternatives, we agreed to set up an epidural injection in hopes that it would alleviate some of the pain and help her ability to walk. Since she had type II diabetes and hypertension, my mother needed to increase her mobility as a means to control her weight and improve her blood sugars and pressure. I later discovered that DISH is thought to be a variant of osteoarthritis (which runs in our family), and is linked to adult onset diabetes (also in the family), the hypothesis being that prolonged insulin production would trigger new bone growth. The past was catching up with us.

~ ★ ~

Over time certain patients will return to the clinic, like Monarch butterflies needing a rest, for a therapeutic tune-up. With the majority of them it is quite difficult not to become attached to their endearing personalities, and as we work together we end up discussing all the recent changes in their lives. One such patient, Father Tim, was an eighty-year-old Catholic priest with a colorful past as a missionary in South America who had a taste for bourbon and a vocabulary like a longshoreman. Although my firm, stiff fingers and deep acupressure and myofascial release treatments helped him manage his lumbosacral muscle spasms, his battle against spinal stenosis was becoming more labored. He knew all the tricks—knee to chest stretches, walking with a pelvic tilt, and pacing his activities so he could rest his spine frequently in a flexed position—in fact, he even went so far as to walk only uphill at his retirement community before calling the attendant to come and pick him up so that he could be spared the jarring pace and extended spinal position of strolling back down. Despite all his efforts, he needed my help more and more frequently as he pondered the wisdom of a undergoing a series of epidural injections.

It had been an incredibly busy week. Patients were on edge in the remaining days before Thanksgiving and were running continually late, their minds fixed on the treats and stresses to come. So, when I arrived and checked my schedule, I was pleased to see the name of my old friend Father Tim listed right before lunch. "Tim, how wonderful to see you," I exclaimed as I worked my way into his treatment room.

"Hey there, Anne, how goes it?" he responded. "My back is killing me! I need a little of your Brünhilde action on my aching butt. I was doing fine until I tried racing Father Clark up and down the hills of San Francisco over the weekend, but now I'm all locked up."

I quickly assessed his spinal range of motion, made sure he had no new neurological signs, and then palpated his lumbar paraspinal muscles. Sure enough, he was as tight as a marine's mattress all through his low back and also in the proximal gluteal and piriformis muscles on both sides of his buttocks. But how was I to manually treat him without exacerbating his pain? In the past I had made sure he was propped up over at least two pillows in prone to prevent his spine from extending and further pinching his already squeezed nerves. I decided that today, we should try some deep tissue mobilization while he lay on his side with his knees pulled in toward his chest. He affirmed, "Yeah, that's the ticket—I can only sleep on my side anyway, so let's try it."

Father Tim arranged himself on his side on the treatment table, and I stood in front of him in the harbor between his chest and knees, thinking that in this position I could block a potential fall forward as I reached across him to press on his back. As I began to orient myself to his rigid back muscles, I felt him begin to shake with laughter. Still palpating (something I could frequently perform, and sometimes still do, with my eyes closed) I absently said, "What's the joke, Father Tim?" Then, I felt it. A firm, overly familiar, answering pressure . . .

"Must you?" I asked, as he dissolved into gales of laughter, still squeezing my rump under his calloused hand. I gripped his trunk in reply with one hand as he was on the verge of laughing himself clear off the table, while I extricated my right buttock from his grasp with the other.

"I feel heaps better already!" He snickered as I fixed him in my 'I am a health professional not to be trifled with' glare. Honestly. After he wiped away his tears of mirth, I tried to maintain my composure and treated him the normal way with soft tissue mobilization, relaxing modalities, and a review of his lumbar flexion-biased exercise regimen. As I left the clinic for lunch and walked toward my car, I suddenly focused on my American Physical Therapy Association–sanctioned license plate frame, which declared "Physical Therapy— The Healing Touch." Who would have thought that a therapist's buttocks could be so therapeutic?

At the time of the incident I had felt completely taken aback and didn't know what to think or how to react, but as I thought about the episode further I realized that this was actually an unexpected form of sexual harassment. Although therapists are used to laying their hands on patients every day, it is always with the patient's consent and with therapeutic intent, and the patient is at free will to end the encounter at any time. Inappropriate touching must never be allowed.

~ ★ ~

Mattie raised herself stiffly from the waiting room chair by thrusting her hips forward as if she were pregnant. Once standing, she staggered to the countertop in the reception area and clutched the edge with a groan and a wince. As I invited her to follow me to a treatment room, she slowly propelled herself along the walls, dragging her right leg with every step. Her physical therapy prescription simply read "Low Back Pain—Evaluate and Treat," but she looked as if she had recently emerged from a full body cast. I watched Mattie's progress through narrowed eyes, wondering if she had suffered nerve damage at some point.

When we finally attained the treatment room, Mattie settled herself in a waiting chair with a grunt. She rummaged through her capricious handbag, saying "I need a pill; I'm diabetic you know. It's always worse when I'm having my period—oh, and sometimes I just hemorrhage and I can't leave the house. That feeling when a clot 'drops'—I can't go to work or do anything but lie in bed and cry and then my sister has to come and look after me. Is that normal? I have bad endometriosis, you know. And now with my back, I can't even walk . . . my gynecologist thinks the back pain is worse because of all the adhesions, but my back doctor doesn't even believe I have endometriosis. He says that you can't diagnose endometriosis without having surgery to look inside, but I'm sure I have adhesions 'cause I feel them tugging on my guts."

I held up my hand, requesting a moment of silence to get a word in edgewise as I inwardly recoiled from her soliloquy. It was distracting talking to Mattie, as she had a wandering eye—one eye was looking straight at me at the same time the other eye was focused on the oleander bush outside the window. I looked into her attending eye, and tried to redirect her. "When did you first hurt your back? How did you hurt it? How long have you had right leg weakness?"

She replied testily, "My leg is fine. I'm trying to tell you, it's my back that hurts!" I sighed inwardly, and began the evaluation. Mattie's lumbar range of motion was nonexistent, as she refused to bend or move her back in any way but resolutely held on to the wall without moving, her face contorted in pain. Manual muscle testing of her lower extremities was also inconclusive, as she would not try to resist my restraining hand when I attempted to assess her leg strength. I noticed that even though she refused to resist my pressure, she was able to fully extend her knee while sitting, indicating that her sciatic nerve was not painful when in a position of tension. Deep tendon reflexes were normal in response to my rubber hammer wielding; since it's nearly impossible to dampen your own reflexes, I could cross this sign off the list. Mattie reported intact sensation with no numbness or tingling in her legs.

After a verbal wrestling match, Mattie consented to lie gingerly supine on the treatment table so that I could test the freedom of her leg movements. I made every effort to move slowly and to forewarn her about how I intended to move her legs before I did so, but I felt nothing but resistance from her regardless of her leg position. She cried out when I flexed her hip to a 90-degree angle, a curious finding since she was able to sit in a chair comfortably with her hips bent to the same degree. When I tried to lift her straight legs one at a time to confirm the absence of neural tension, she moaned and cried out in pain, even though the same angles had been pain free when she was seated. Then, I cautiously asked her to turn over so I could feel her back.

Mattie's lower back looked completely normal. I warily touched her, talking all the while so as not to cause alarm, but she shuddered as my fingers made contact with butterfly-kiss lightness. Then, she groaned in appreciation, "The only thing that helps me feel better is massage." This was a red flag statement, if I'd ever heard one. Was she legitimate, or was she a malingerer? I could feel no areas of increased soft tissue density in her back muscles and soft tissues, and no evidence of muscle spasms or tightness. I decided to treat her as actively as possible in order to help her regain her independence—too much passive therapy with massage and modalities like ultrasound could create a needy monster.

Three days later, Mattie's name appeared on my schedule for a second visit. The patient preceding her had canceled, so I happened to be sitting at the front desk charting on the morning's patients when she arrived. The clinic faces a courtyard containing a fountain, and as our patients approach, we can see them through the windows as they make their way toward our doors. Amazingly, Mattie was walking without the trace of a limp, animatedly talking with the sister who had accompanied her on the previous visit. They opened the door, and Mattie was once again reduced to a cringing, limping shadow of her former self. My earlier hunch was confirmed—she was a malingerer. This observation sealed her fate. Active therapeutic exercise is the only cure for this condition, and over subsequent visits I made her work hard. Each time she would ask for a massage, but I explained that since research shows that active exercise was the method of treatment most likely to resolve her terrible pain, that was to be our emphasis. Miraculously, with this approach Mattie rapidly lost her limp and disappeared from the schedule, never to be seen again.

~ ★ ~

The decision about which continuing education course to attend at any given time depends on a variety of factors. I am usually drawn to courses that are close by (since I hate traveling), offered by a renowned expert (so that I'm not wasting my time), and that cover material I have not recently reviewed (to refresh my memory and skills). One particular lumbar spine course stands out in my mind as an especially singular experience.

Two other PTs from the large outpatient clinic where I worked had decided to drive one hundred miles to attend a weekend course on lumbar dysfunction with an internationally acclaimed clinician, and decided to split a hotel room. Although I usually prefer to stay closer to home in order to offset the expense of a hotel, this expert's reputation was such that I was encouraged to attend anyway. We arose in the predawn hours and carpooled to the course in my colleague's Toyota, trading clinic horror stories and difficult case reports as we went. When we reached the parking lot of our sister clinic, we toasted each other with mimosas in plastic champagne flutes before entering the building. I would never consider imbibing alcohol before laying my hands upon another person, but day one of this course was meant to be a lecture, so I felt free to enjoy the camaraderie with my colleagues. There were muffins and coffee available to sop up the alcohol in our bloodstreams as we sat down to listen to the first theoretical part of the course. That afternoon, our esteemed expert changed his format and we were asked to split off and apply our newfound knowledge to each other's spines. Fortunately, by this time the mimosas had long been metabolized. My two colleagues decided to work together, so I made a new friend with whom to practice spinal mobilization techniques.

As always, each therapist had brought a large towel to lie on, and we were attired in "lab clothes," which in my case consisted of loose-fitting khaki shorts and a black full-coverage sports bra beneath a favorite old purple T-shirt. Laboratory assistants circulated around the room to offer the participating therapists feedback about correct hand placement and technique. My lab partner, Angela, and I were enjoying the review of palpation of lumbar spinal landmarks, when she decided to excuse herself to use the restroom. Temporarily without a partner, I relaxed on our treatment table and observed the other therapists practicing on each other. It was during this interlude that one of the lab assistants approached my table and stood behind me for a moment or two. Then, he leaned forward and whispered into my ear, "You're too young to be this fat." Startled, I whipped around to look at him, thinking I had misheard. "What did you just say?" I asked.

"You should be in better shape, that's all," he explained.

I was speechless. As he drifted off to another table, my thoughts boiled and surged. What nerve! What right did he have to comment on my size? He was partially bald—was that a preferable condition to being heavy? Besides, at an active five foot eight inches and sporting a reasonable weight on my medium-sized frame, I didn't feel obese.

As my lab partner returned, I asked, "Hey Angela, has that assistant guy talked to you yet?"

"Yeah, he gave me some input about my body mechanics earlier when you were getting a cup of coffee. Why?"

Never mind. Angela was shorter and had a good twenty pounds on me, yet had emerged unscathed from her conversation with him. Was this one of those schoolyard scenarios, where the boy pulls the pigtails and taunts the little girl he has a crush on? But I was married, and wearing a ring . . . it just didn't make any sense. I decided to try to let it go, but felt disturbed and vaguely hurt for a long time afterward. The memory of the incident resurfaced on occasion, serving as a reminder of the powers of communication—sometimes, casual comments that may seem innocuous at the time can have a lasting impact on others, and I resolved to pay closer attention to my own remarks.

~ ★ ~

I was standing at the desk, completing my charts when Tad finally arrived. He was twenty minutes late for his initial evaluation, a circumstance that throws my schedule into a tailspin since I see a patient every thirty minutes without fail. It is always a dilemma to decide what to do—should I try to complete an initial assessment, knowing that I would run behind schedule and inconvenience the other patients all day long? Should I perform a "quick and dirty" evaluation, focusing on the highlights of his condition and then at least get him started with some aspects of treatment? Or, should I ask him to reschedule to another day or later the same day with another therapist, giving him time to fill out his paper-work and relax for a short while?

Glancing down at the old-fashioned appointment book, I noticed that there were no openings later on. By this time, Tad had painfully negotiated his way across the short distance from the door, and was leaning heavily on the desk with a pinched expression, rivulets of sweat running in front of his ears that stuck out like the handles of a loving cup. I had to do something for the poor guy and was unable to turn him away without at least offering him some respite. I smiled at him, and accepted his prescription which read, "Status Post L4/5 and L5/S1 PLIF—Evaluate and Treat." Inwardly I sighed; posterior lumbar interbody fusions were tricky things that were usually extremely painful to recover from, and even then, some patients never regained their previous activity levels. Poor Tad—I hoped he would be one of the lucky ones.

We navigated the short hallway together in silence, Tad's concentration com-pletely focused on pushing his rolling walker forward in a supreme effort to stand upright. As we entered the treatment room, he slid laboriously into a chair without altering his tense posture. I nipped out to get him a paper cup full of water as he looked all-in and I didn't want him to faint. He drank, and then offered me a shaky smile. "It's hard to believe how much effort that took! I thought it would be much easier to get here; after all, just step from the truck onto the elevator and down a short hallway . . . but man, I'm beat!"

"So, what happened—how did you hurt yourself?" I asked.

"You should see the other guy," he replied wryly. "I'm a sheriff, and in the heat of the chase I had to launch myself over a fence and drop down into someone's backyard to get the bad guy. Unfortunately, after I scaled the fence the drop was quite a bit steeper than either one of us had thought, so I ended up landing on top of him! He broke his ribs and shoulder and I heard a big 'pop' in my back when I fell, but I was able to restrain him. I went through a bunch of therapy, but nothing worked. Finally they did an MRI, and it turned out that two discs were sitting on my nerves and my spine had shifted and was really unstable. It was a spondi . . . a spondylo . . . I can't remember the right word, but my spine slipped. So, surgery was the only cure and here I am to recover; and I can hardly wait to get out of this clamshell," he said as he knocked on the hard plastic back brace hidden beneath his T-shirt.

"You probably mean a spondylolisthesis," I said.

"Yup, that's it," he replied.

"Did you use your own bone in-between the vertebrae, or did you get some from the bone bank?" I asked.

"They used cadaver bone, which they stuck into one of those titanium cages after getting rid of my crapped-out discs," he said. "Then, they put me back together with plates and screws to keep stuff from shifting around . . . but I still feel like Humpty Dumpty."

Tad's neurosurgeon wanted him to wear the hard brace for at least four months, but depending on how well Tad's back fused, it could take longer. Over the months ahead his progress would be tracked on X-ray to be sure the bones were starting to meld together. Fortunately, Tad wasn't a huge guy and had been given the OK by his surgeon to remove his brace briefly to shower and for certain aspects of therapy. I began by carefully testing his leg strength (quite weak, no wonder that he needed to use the walker), reflexes, sensation, and neural tension. Tad's neural signs were all good, and his primary problem was trunk and leg weakness and continuing pain, for which he was taking narcotics. This was not unusual, as most spine surgeons try to avoid using nonsteroidal anti-inflammatory medications for pain control following fusions since the drugs tend to inhibit bone healing. Any narcotic dependence would have to be dealt with later. Tad's incision was about six inches long, beefy red, and fresh. I could feel that he had severe muscle spasms throughout his thoracic and lumbar area covered by a large pool of swelling in the small of his back, like submerged trees lurking beneath a lake surface. We had a lot of work to do.

The lumbar spine is intimately supported and strengthened by strong abdominal muscles, which act like a natural corset to protect and prevent unwanted movement. After surgery Tad's stomach muscles had shut down completely, offering him no natural support, so that despite the restrictive presence of his brace Tad was constantly at risk of blowing out his fusion. We began carefully with lower extremity stretching exercises in supine to indirectly lengthen and relax the tight lumbosacral muscles through the gluteal and hip muscles, and moved on to myofascial release and gentle soft tissue mobilization of the lumbar paraspinals to reduce his guarding spasms. We immediately explored proper body mechanics so as to spare him additional movement to the spine and help keep things quiet while he healed, and progressed to working on strengthening his sleeping abdominal muscles.

One day, Tad greeted me with a sheepish look on his face and a burning question on his lips. He was still wearing the clamshell brace, but now he was moving around without the walker, although he had extremely poor endurance and needed to lean on a cane for support. He wasn't able to look me in the eye. "Hey, I was just wondering what guys like me do after this kind of surgery," he began. "Are there any safe, you know, *positions* that I can be in with my girlfriend?"

I had read somewhere that more than 80 percent of surgeons are loathe to discuss sexual issues with their patients, and when they do, more than 95 percent of them spend five minutes or less on the topic; therefore, I always tend to assume that most patients are in the dark as to when and how to proceed. For this purpose, I keep a professional booklet nearby that I can give to patients and clinically discuss which positions might aggravate their condition. This piece of patient education is especially important for patient with low back disorders, as often it is critical that they maintain a position of lumbar neutral, mild flexion, or extension (depending on the underlying diagnosis), in order to protect their underlying fusion, stenosis, or disc problem. Although the booklet is helpful, embarrassment is still common as we go over the line drawings depicting couples performing intercourse in various ways, circling the positions that theoretically might be considered "safe" for the individual patient.

In Tad's case, he was definitely advised to clear this form of exercise first with his neurosurgeon before going ahead. Once cleared for sexual activity, he would have to continue wearing his brace to protect his healing lumbar spinal fusion while otherwise engaged. Throughout rehabilitation patients are repeatedly instructed in self-awareness of their body mechanics and back position in order to protect the healing spine, but most people are simply unable to retain objectivity in the midst of a heated encounter and must rely upon sensible positioning, corsets or braces, and a sensitive partner. Fortunately, Tad was motivated and in a stable relationship, and so was able to explore this necessary return to normalcy without incident.

Over our subsequent visits, the wild, embarrassed look in his eye was replaced by a calm determination to get better. He admitted that he had been extremely nervous about bringing up the topic of sex during our physical therapy session, but had been feeling so inadequate with his fiancée that he was empowered to stumble on and ask me about it. "After all, therapists can be more approachable than neurosurgeons," he explained with a grateful smile.

~ ★ ~

Regardless of the person's diagnosis, physical condition, or attitude, I strive to be approachable and to put my patients at ease. Most of the time this is appreciated, but on occasion I wonder if I am able to get through at all to some patients.

When I initially met Sally, a beautifully dressed woman in her late sixties with a fine manicure and perfect permanent wave, the first thing I noticed was her ugly posture. Her medical history included chronic back strain and a small, old L1 compression fracture, and she told me that she had been experiencing low back pain for about ten years.

"Sally, what activities or positions do you notice aggravate your low back pain?" I asked.

"Nothing special—it always hurts," she replied.

"Well, do you notice that the pain is worse by the end of the day, or is it worse first thing in the morning?" I persisted.

"It hurts all the time, but gets worse by evening," she said.

I requested that she rate her pain on a scale of zero to ten, zero being no pain at all and ten being the worst pain she could imagine, pain so intense that she would need to call an ambulance and go to the hospital right away. Sally coolly responded, "It's a nine."

"Is it always a nine?" I asked. "You don't look too uncomfortable right now . . . or do you mean that by tonight it will feel that strong?"

"By tonight it'll be a ten," she replied placidly.

I took her pulse and blood pressure, which were both normal. She wasn't breathing fast, had no evidence of sweating or distress, and quite frankly didn't have a hair out of place. Nine out of ten? I think not.

I asked, "What does your typical day look like? Are you working or volunteering? Do you like to go for walks? Read? Go shopping?"

"I'm retired, and I like to watch TV," she said.

"Oh, I see—do you have a favorite program, or do you kind of watch here and there throughout the day?" I asked.

"I like the soap operas," she said. "*All My Children* is my favorite, but I watch them all. Then, I work my way through the game shows. By nightfall, my back is really sore."

My back would be sore too, after sitting and watching television all day long! It turned out that once Sally had retired from work ten years previously, she retired from life. All day and most of the night she was glued to her beloved TV set, getting up only to fix herself and her husband the occasional sandwich or bowl of soup. To make matters worse, she cocooned herself in a ramshackle, soft old sofa and slumped away her time there. I began treatment by loosening up her rigid thoracolumbar paraspinals with soft tissue mobilization techniques, then showed her how to correct her sitting posture and pace her television viewing activities, changing seats from time to time. I asked her to reposition and stretch during the commercial breaks so that she could give her muscles much-needed respite from slumping against gravity without missing any of the action onscreen.

During the following treatment session with Sally, I asked how the exercises and position changes were going. "I haven't tried them yet," she replied. Too frustrating; most patients who report nine out of ten levels of pain are willing to try anything to make it better. Again I reiterated the importance of treating her body more kindly, and suggested that she at least use a supportive lumbar cushion to help her low back stay more comfortable through the hours of slumping on the sofa. I showed her how to use a piece of elastic Thera-Band® tied to a nearby doorknob or chair to exercise during commercials to help increase the circulation of blood to her tight muscles and engage better posture. I found out that she had a heating pad, and asked that she use it on her tight paraspinal muscles before her pain went from a "nine to a ten."

Each time I saw her, Sally reported no changes in her lumbar pain despite all my suggestions and manual therapy techniques. She also reported complete noncompliance with the exercises, stretches, postural changes, and ergonomic suggestions. After a few sessions, we agreed to part ways; Sally simply didn't want to bother, and I was unable to reach her in a meaningful way.

The Keystone in the Arch

It is more important to know what sort of person has a disease than to know what sort of disease a person has.

—*Hippocrates of Kos, Greek physician (460 BC–370 BC)*

The sacrum is the last functional "vertebra" of the spine. Consisting of between four and six fused vertebrae, it is the keystone within the arch of the pelvis that connects the spine to the hips. The anatomical location where the spine attaches to the pelvis, the sacroiliac (SI) joint, enjoys a love-hate relationship with the medical community at large. Because of the SI joint's irregular shape and its tendency to fuse with aging, many health professionals feel that the sacroiliac is inert and unable to move. Others think that the SI joint is able to glide slightly along its irregular, C-shaped surface in response to injury, trauma, or hormonal fluctuations, producing a mechanically based pain.

The SI joint's purpose is to dissipate loading forces from the spine and upper body through to the pelvic base and lower extremities. At the same time, the joint also absorbs some of the shock produced from ground reaction force, acting as a barrier between the floor and the spine. Asymmetrical forces that repeatedly impact the SI joint can cause pain and dysfunction, including those caused by uneven leg length, leg weakness, unilateral muscle tightness, or stretched support ligaments. Women especially have an increased risk of SI joint pain due to pelvic ligamentous laxity that occurs with hormonal fluctuations each month and during pregnancy. In the clinic, a proportion of patients with a diagnosis of lumbar pain may actually be experiencing a problem with the sacroiliac joint that is furtively lurking under the radar and may have "failed" previous attempts at physical therapy.

~ ★ ~

I had been happily seeing patients at my colleague's small outpatient clinic for a few years and had gotten to know some of the regulars who had suffered from recurring misfortune when I first met Gerry. One of Jack's usual patients, Gerry had been struggling for a long time with stiffness following her total knee replacement. Because her right knee had formed adhesions that served to effectively glue the knee into a rigid position, she was unable to drive and had to be transported to the clinic three times a week via the gallant chauffeuring efforts of her husband. Over a period of months, I had seen Gerry gradually win her battle over the sticky scar tissue as she limped past me on her way to see Jack. Therapy to stretch her knee was a slow, tortured process during which she was frequently discouraged; however, there was no other path to regaining her flexibility. Severely osteoporotic, she could not safely undergo a manipulation under anesthesia, the process in which the patient is anesthetized to allow the surgeon to literally force the knee into flexion and extension. This brutal but necessary manipulation technique effectively breaks the adhesions apart with a thunderous crack, but in Gerry's case, the risk of her bones breaking before the adhesions might surrender was very real.

After many sequential treatment successes, Gerry had finally achieved the majority of her expected knee flexibility and gone on her merry way. Then, months later, I saw her name on my schedule to be evaluated for low back pain. Jack's schedule was full, and she wanted to be seen as soon as possible. When she finally arrived, Gerry showed no trace of her former limp but instead had a very short, shuffling stride length. When she saw me she grimaced, "It's my back now; it just won't go away! I've tried hot pads and even acupuncture, but I can't get any relief. We're supposed to travel and see our family back East next month, but I may have to cancel it—I just can't get around that easily."

We slowly reached the privacy of a treatment room together after an agonizing journey down the short hallway. Once we had safely closed the door, I asked Gerry to point out where the pain was; in response, she brushed her hand across her lower back in an impatient sweeping gesture. "If you could put one finger on the spot that hurts, where would you point?" I asked insistently. This time, Gerry pointed to the small dimple at the right side of her lower back. This spot overlays the right posterior superior iliac spine (PSIS), and correlates with one half of the sacroiliac joint. The dimple marks one of the paired spots in the lumbosacral region that is known to be a tender point for sacroiliac dysfunction. Already my suspicions were building. After testing her general lumbar spine range of motion (normal), I assessed her sacroiliac movement. This can be done in several ways, but I started with the march, flare, and side bending tests.

For the march test, Gerry turned her back to me and slowly marched in place with her knees coming up high as I sat behind her and palpated the movement of her PSIS bony landmarks for symmetry. To examine flare, I had Gerry, while still standing, move one foot in and out from midline while keeping her heels planted firmly on the ground as I palpated the degree of movement of her pelvis at each anterior superior iliac spine (ASIS). Finally, I assessed the extent of sacral motion by simultaneously palpating the left and right sacral surfaces as Gerry moved slowly into a position of left and then right side bending. Sure enough, she was completely jammed up on the right, with very little relative motion occurring on that side. To gather more information, I asked her to lie supine on the treatment table.

"The other problem I'm having is that I think my knee replacement is the wrong size," she said. "I've noticed that one leg seems a lot longer than the other—do you think my orthopedic surgeon made a mistake? I guess it could certainly account for my back pain."

She had a point. Despite popular belief, surgeons are human beings too and some are more particular with their work than others, which can result in the occasional asymmetry. However, I knew the work of her surgeon well and had observed him in action in the operating room—he was known for his carefulness, accuracy, and caution, so in her case I thought that error was unlikely. To check, I asked her to briefly lift her hips up in the air, and then set them down again on the treatment table to reset her position. I then gently brought her legs down into extension. Sure enough, her right leg appeared to be nearly two inches shorter than her left. A true leg length discrepancy can be the result of a naturally longer/shorter femur or tibia, but it can also be caused by a too-large hip or knee prosthesis or a leg being shortened too much under the hands of an overzealous surgeon who accidentally removes too much bone before implanting the prosthesis. However, the legs may also appear to be unequal when the pelvis is unlevel.

Asking Gerry not to move, I whipped out my tape measure to perform the quick clinical test for assessing true leg length differences. Although the most accurate method of comparing leg lengths is by X-ray, the direct tape measure method has sufficient reliability when performed in a consistent manner.

With one end of my tape measure held firmly at Gerry's ASIS, I extended the tape measure down her leg to end at the medial malleolus. After repeating this exercise on the other leg, I found that her legs were roughly the same length, increasing my suspicions that her pelvis might be out of position. I then palpated her bony pelvic landmarks, looking at the orientation of her bones in relationship to midline and to each other. Sure enough, her landmarks were asymmetrical, indicating a pelvis that had shifted not only front-to-back (ilial rotation), but also side-to-side (ilial inflare/outflare).

The most likely cause of Gerry's apparent leg length discrepancy and SI joint asymmetry was limping around for all those months with her stiff knee, each step relentlessly pushing uneven forces into her pelvis. Fortunately, pelvic asymmetry can be normalized by physical therapy treatment that involves the use of muscle energy techniques, which can mobilize the joint back into position through isometric muscle contractions of selected leg muscles. By fixing the legs in specific positions and then asking the patient to generate a muscle contraction while the therapist restricts actual movement, the pelvis can subtly be shifted back into a symmetrical position.

Gerry and I proceeded to resist each other's movements as I placed her legs into optimal positions to influence her pelvis. Then, I asked her to squeeze her knees together onto my clenched hands in order to reset the disc at the pubis symphysis, located at the anterior pelvis. With each mobilization, Gerry's ability to squeeze became stronger and less painful, a good sign that she was returning to symmetry, since, when the muscles are placed in an overly shortened or lengthened position, they are unable to perform to their best ability and will respond with a feeling of strain.

When I reassessed her bony landmarks, Gerry's pelvis was back in balance and her legs looked even once more. "It's amazing!" she cried when she stood up. "I feel like I'm standing straight again." I reviewed the need for her to activate her abdominal muscles and to move in a symmetrical manner, because, since she had been hobbling around unevenly for many months, there was a risk that her SI joint would "remember" being out of position and naturally want to gravitate back to its painful asymmetrical position.

~ ★ ~

The path to getting accepted into physical therapy school is a long, tortuous one. With the aging of the baby boomers (a group to which I can claim membership), physical therapy has become one of the most hotly sought-after professions; in some states, getting accepted into PT school is far more difficult than getting into medical school. In my case, I had returned to graduate school as an "older" student, having spent a number of years working in medical research. The years of research were satisfying, but over time I craved helping people more directly than I could by discovering a few small pieces of the puzzle over months' and years' time. Once I decided to go back to school for my master's degree in physical therapy, I wanted to be accepted into the excellent graduate program at UCSF/SFSU. Although I had been working for many years at UCSF in the Cardiovascular Research Institute, the graduate program in physical therapy was completely separate, so my chances of admission were the same as everyone else's. Nonetheless, I felt such a growing certainty within me that I would be accepted into this school that I foolishly refused to apply anywhere else.

This calculated risk required that I take eight additional prerequisite courses at SFSU while continuing to work full-time on the research projects, study for the Graduate Record Examination, and find the time to put in more than 150 hours volunteering in a variety of physical therapy clinics to prove my intent. It was a full schedule, but I was driven with the certainty of my destiny. To this day it remains unclear whether my driven, obsessive nature is a benefit or a curse; although it spurs me to achieve more and more, it has also gotten me into trouble. One incident that I painfully remember, for example, is pushing myself to ride the Davis Double Century bicycle race on a last-minute bet, for which I forced my poor, untrained body to pedal two hundred miles within twenty hours without respite—all for a pizza!

I threw myself into the prerequisite coursework at SFSU with my usual zeal, weathering the 1989 Loma Prieta earthquake while in class (amazing to watch the floor flow past my safe spot in the classroom doorway in waves, the seemingly solid tile instantly transformed into liquid) and soaking up the formaldehyde fumes and Latin anatomical terms with curiosity and a sense of wonder. In the end, it was my fanatical approach and attention to detail that earned me the extra credit point on the anatomy lab practical exam. Each station was carefully arranged with either a dismembered limb, a microscope, or a bone to be identified within the allotted two minutes, at which point you had to move on to the next station whether you had decided on your answer or not. In this instance, I was happily labeling my answer sheet with confidence until I reached station number 34, the pelvic X-ray. The tag read: "Identify if this is a male or a female pelvis. Extra credit: write in what you see as being especially different on this plain film." I squinted at the light box, remembering that the male pelvis is more upright than the female one, which flares out in a butterfly-like shape with laterally placed hip sockets. The clock was ticking, and as I struggled to make up my mind I leaned closer to the light box. Before I had even fully processed it, I blinked in disbelief and looked up to see my anatomy instructor grinning at me. I checked the X-ray again, and there it was—the faint, delicate outline of a baby's skeleton tucked inside the definitely female pelvis.

~ ★ ~

In the process of assessing the pelvis, physical therapists sometimes get closer than they would like to other people's "personal" areas. At this point I have pretty much seen it all, but at times I have been momentarily taken aback by the lack of modesty or the singular personal taste in undergarments. During these times it is my job to refrain from reacting or commenting, but just to keep my attention on the task at hand. It can be difficult.

Genevieve had requested a female therapist to help her with her bursitis problem, so she fell onto my schedule, the only other therapist in the clinic being male. She was a native Frenchwoman and was an opinionated artist with a booming, sonorous voice. Her shock of kinky, curly hair sprang away unfettered from both her head and her armpits, and her expressive features were unencumbered by makeup. As soon as she saw me enter the room she stood and pulled up her skirt to reveal a lacy black thong, and began to pull apart her buttocks before the door had even closed behind me. "The problem is here," she insisted, as she traced her fingers along her left seat bone. "Look! Can you see? This spot," she said, jabbing at her nether regions and bending forward. I peered at her bottom, seeing nothing more alarming than the slender frilly line of the thong disappearing between her legs.

"Why don't you get comfortable for a moment—would you like to put on a gown?" I suggested.

"Oh, no, I'm fine," Genevieve maintained. "You are also a woman, and I am a woman, and everything is the same between us, no? We are both relaxed among ourselves."

For fear of making a fuss about her state of undress and embarrassing her, I acquiesced and began to assess her problem. She described left seat bone pain when sitting, especially on hard surfaces, and was having trouble working on her sculptures, since her method required her to spend a great deal of time sitting on the floor in the tailor-sit position while working with her clay. My expression cleared as I visualized her work position. "Ah, you have 'weaver's bottom'!" I explained. "This condition was common around the time of the Industrial Revolution, especially in trades that required workers such as weavers and tailors to make repeated forward and backward rocking movements while sitting on hard surfaces for long periods of time. All that moving around on the seat bones would repeatedly squeeze the ischial bursa between the gluteus maximus muscle attachments and the seat bone, which is also known as the ischial tuberosity. The bursa is supposed to act as a cushion to reduce friction between the muscles and the bones, but once it gets inflamed, it causes a lot of pain to the sitter."

I find that the seat bone is most easily palpated in the supine position, so I asked Genevieve to lie on her back and bend her left knee toward her chest. Sure enough, when I palpated her left ischial tuberosity I could feel a dense, thickened area underneath my finger pads. "That's it!" she agreed, convulsively kicking out in her discomfort. From that point on, treatment was relatively simple: ultrasound, interferential stimulation, and soft tissue mobilization over the bursa to increase blood flow and speed the healing process; stretching of tight gluteal and hamstring muscles crossing the area to reduce friction across the inflamed bursa; and strict instructions to sit on padded surfaces to avoid compression of the supremely irritated tissues. Genevieve was a very compliant and motivated patient, sculpting being both her passion and her career. She was also perceptive—the next time I saw her, the thong was gone and she was wearing a pair of peach-colored tap pants beneath her skirt.

~ ★ ~

I once jarred my own SI joint by using an asymmetrical breaststroke kick while relaxing in the pool on holiday, and spent hours on the floor asking my husband, "Is my left hip bone higher than the right? Does my sacrum look rotated? Can you see if my right leg is shorter?" as he bemusedly poked around my bony pelvic landmarks with his thumbs. Sacroiliac asymmetry can easily happen with all sorts of conditions, but is especially common with pregnancy. The hormonal changes that allow for the eventual softening and stretching of pelvic ligaments can render women unstable in their SI joints, and they must sometimes resort to using sacroiliac belts and other external supports to stabilize their grinding bones just to be able to hobble around. One of the best forms of stabilizing a wandering SI joint is abdominal activation, but this becomes increasingly difficult with the ever-expanding stomach of pregnancy.

Ellen first came in for treatment several years ago, after the birth of her second child. She had suffered with radiating right sciatica that originated from her low back during her last trimester, and despite a successful recovery after delivering her daughter, the sciatica stubbornly remained. Her team of physicians had identified a sloppy bulging lumbar disc at L5/S1, the last level above the sacrum, and had eventually performed intradiscal electrothermal therapy (IDET) on the faulty disc to help shrink and toughen it. The IDET procedure is a minimally invasive intervention in which the surgeon passes a small wire into the disc, and then using radiofrequency technology electrically heats the injured disc, which seals any cracks or tears and reduces disc sensitivity. In Ellen's case, although the surgery had gone well and her sciatica was gone, her back pain remained. When I saw Ellen to help her strengthen her abdominals and trunk muscles after the IDET procedure, she was unable to sit down or lift her baby and felt she had to keep moving around to alleviate the pain. She was especially anxious at the thought of returning to work, as she felt incapable of sitting at her computer for the required eight hours each day. In desperation, Ellen had convinced her doctor to perform a repeat MRI, thinking that she had reruptured her disc, but the imaging test had revealed that all was well. Time was running out before she had to return to work or possibly lose her job.

In the course of my assessment of her back pain, I noticed that Ellen's abdominal muscles were still slack and inactive following childbirth and that she was unable to stabilize her body in space. I asked her to stand before me in a relaxed way and applied a gentle force to one of her shoulders. She swayed violently, nearly staggering to keep her balance, and pointed to her right SI joint in pain. Then I asked her to pull her tummy muscles in to the best of her abilities, and reapplied my light force to her shoulder. No pain. Her face lit up. "Is that all I have to do?" she asked in excitement. But it was not to be so simple, as her SI joint was twisted every which way. I put her through the clinical movement tests for SI dysfunction and found that she failed them all, revealing multiplanar asymmetry. Despite having healed well from her IDET procedure, Ellen's pelvis was well and truly stuck.

I set about rebalancing her SI joint using the isometric muscle energy techniques, and with each mobilization she grew more able to resist my pressure. Finally, after we worked our way through each aspect of this three-dimensional joint, I asked her to stand up and walk back and forth in the treatment room a few steps. Ellen's mouth dropped open, and she said with delight, "My back feels weightless! I have no pain . . . let me try sitting down." She eased into the chair, and relaxed her spine carefully against the back of the chair. "So far, so good . . . I'm cured!" I hastened to explain to her that with all the directions her SI joint had slipped into, it might not recognize a symmetrical position for some time. She would have to begin a strict daily regimen of abdominal activation exercises to help "hold" the joint in balance. She eagerly absorbed all my advice like a sponge, and rushed off to get started.

Over the succeeding months, I saw Ellen only occasionally. She was one of the most motivated patients I had, only coming back for a tune-up if she had inadvertently twisted or moved in the wrong way. Each time Ellen returned, I found that she was increasingly self-aware. She would come in saying, "I think my sacrum is twisted to the left," or "my right hip feels rotated back," and I would perform the clinical tests and palpate her bony landmarks to confirm that she was correct in her own assessment. Her backsliding occurred less and less as she gradually strengthened her abdominal muscles, until finally I needed to see her only once a year after her summer vacation. Ellen was always especially active on vacation, and in the course of walking along the Great Wall of China or learning how to windsurf, her SI joint would briefly misbehave. If it was September, it was time to see Ellen.

~ ★ ~

One of the most important things we can do to help keep our sacroiliac joints and lumbar spines healthy and quiet is to perform routine lower abdominal strengthening exercises. Unfortunately, these exercises are the ugly stepsisters of the fitness world, as they are relatively dull, repetitive, and uninspiring, and are typically abandoned at the first sign of a pain-free lumbopelvic area. However, "normal" exercises such as Tai Chi, yoga, and even horseback riding may become a more palatable substitute, as these activities can still challenge the all-important core trunk muscles in a much more entertaining way. Every year when I see my doctor for my annual checkup, she comments on the strength of my abdominals, claiming that she can barely palpate through the muscles to feel the organs beneath. Do I have six-pack abs? No. Do I spend hours each day in the gym? No. I simply tighten my lower abdominal muscles thousands of times a day as I give my patients resistance, click the pins in and out of the exercise equipment, and push the treatment carts containing the electrical stimulation and ultrasound units around. Of course, it helps that I ride my horse at speed several times a week—stabilizing my body on the moving surface of a horse provides a great abdominal activation challenge.

~ ★ ~

The weak winter sunlight forced its way between the slats of the blinds, slashing across Joe's face like the white ribs depicted on a chest X-ray. As he stood up, the light strands fell away and his pained expression became apparent. Joe winced unwillingly and blurted, "Pardon my fat ass—it's been killing me." A local police officer, Joe had been having increasing amounts of low back, pelvis, and hip pain that was beginning to interfere with his job. One of the biggest problems was his gun belt, a bulky leather extravagance that he had to wear at all times, even when sitting in his cruiser. Getting in and out of the car quickly was proving to be a major problem as the pain in his low back and buttocks was aggravated by the resistance of the belt snagging on the door frame. Joe had been unable to success-fully chase down a perpetrator on more than one occasion, and he was beginning to consider leaving the police force to find another, less active job. The trouble was, he loved the job and was one in a long line of police officers in his family. Joe had been treated at another clinic for lumbar strains and sprains, but became only transiently better, the muscle spasms and low back pain returning over and over.

"I'm so stiff in the morning that I'm even having trouble lacing up my boots," Joe complained. "I'm only thirty-three years old, for Christ's sake, and I'm moving around like my Grandpa." Examination of his lumbar spine range of motion revealed minor stiffness in all directions, but especially with forward bend-ing. "You're just a tad bit stiff there," I commented as Joe struggled to reach his fingertips beyond his knees.

"Yeah, heaven help me if I drop my doughnut!" he joked. "But half the time I feel like if I just bend a little bit forward, it helps."

Morning stiffness is one of the signs commonly associated with osteoarthritis, so I asked Joe if he had any family history of arthritis. "Yeah, my Dad had some trouble with his back by the time he was in his forties," he said. Joe's leg strength, reflexes, and sensation were intact, and he had no signs of neural tension. However, I had difficulty bringing his legs up one at a time into the straight leg test position due to the tightness of his hamstring muscles and the stiffness in his hip joints. I had Joe flip over onto his stomach so that I could see and feel his back. His lumbar paraspinal muscles were rigid with spasm, and his gluteal and piriformis muscles were tight and tender. I gently placed my thumbs on his posterior superior iliac spines bilaterally, the typical "hot spots" for sacroiliac pain. Joe shrank into the treatment table to get as far away from me as he could. "Now that hurts!" he exclaimed. Curiously, his pelvic landmarks were mirror images of each other, with no evidence of sacroiliac asymmetry. Joe's lower lumbar spinous and transverse processes were also tender, and stiff in response to my posterior-to-anterior pressures. "Did your doctor ever take any X-rays of your back?" I asked.

"No, right now he thinks it's just a muscle problem and that I just need to get in better shape," Joe responded. "The problem is, I've tried all kinds of things to help me get stronger, but all I feel is stiffer and more tired. Geez, I don't want to end up like my Dad! He just got more and more bent over, and never felt like playing with us."

I flashed on a mental image of a small, elderly Asian man I had seen the previous weekend as I had driven past a church. The man was dressed nicely in a suit and looked as if he wanted to cross the street to go to the church. However, he was hunched over so badly that he had difficulty lifting his head high enough to see the oncoming traffic. He stood on the curb, agonizingly twisting his head from side to side like a turtle poking its head out from the shell as he squinted at the passing cars. I had slowed down and waved at him to encourage him to cross safely in front of my car, but he had impatiently motioned me on. As I pulled away, I looked in my rearview mirror and saw him shuffle slowly and painfully across the street during a gap in the traffic behind me. His stiff, flexed posture was classic for ankylosing spondylitis, an inflammatory arthritis that begins in the SI joints and moves all the way up the spine, eventually freezing the person into one position. The disease has a strong genetic component, and is more commonly found in men.

"Has your doctor done any blood work for you?" I asked.

"No, nothing out of the ordinary," Joe said. We always have a physical at work, but they just look at our blood count and stuff like that and everything's always been fine. Why do you ask?"

"I think it's possible you might have a type of arthritis that specifically affects your pelvis and spine," I said. "But the easiest way to be sure about it is to take an X-ray and do some specific blood tests to look for certain markers."

"Aren't I too young for arthritis?" Joe asked worriedly.

"Not necessarily—there is a genetic component, and some of us are luckier than others regarding whether and how early we might get it," I responded.

I showed Joe how to start specifically working on the tight muscles in his back, hips, and legs as well as how to perform a progression of abdominal activation exercises to help stabilize and support his back and pelvis, cautioning him to keep the strengthening exercises pain free. After some time, Joe returned clutching a large square X-ray folder.

"You were right!" he said. "Look at these—my doctor shot some X-rays and found a bunch of arthritis and inflammation in the low back and sacroiliac joints. In fact, he said my SI joints were in the process of fusing. Based on these, he ordered some blood work and found that I have 'achy-lousy spaghetti' or something like that."

"Do you mean 'ankylosing spondylitis'?" I asked.

"Yeah, that's the one," he said. "The doc said that exercise would help me as long as it's not too strenuous, but that eventually I'll have some decisions to make about work. He said that the condition can literally be a pain in the ass!"

"The biggest thing you'll need to focus on is boring old posture," I said, "because your spine will want to keep getting stiffer in a flexed position like your Dad's did. You need lots of extension exercises to help keep your back straight, plenty of deep breathing exercises to keep your ribs expanded, and no more slumping on the couch with the remote in front of the TV! If you like swimming, that helps with flexibility and general fitness; you're not the kind of guy who should be pounding along on a running track. Oh, and it can also help to sleep on a firm bed, using only a small pillow if you're a back-sleeper, to maintain a straighter spinal position."

Joe followed through. I came across him many years later in a drugstore while picking up a few things, and he looked good. He said that his SI joints and lower spine had fused and were no longer painful, he had a membership to a gym with a swimming pool, and that he was now working in a different division at the police department as a detective. Life was good, and he hadn't become stooped over despite the inexorable pressure of his disease.

~ ★ ~

Health professionals in a variety of settings are rightly accused of having appalling handwriting skills. My own excuse is that we are often in such a hurry we must abbreviate, utilizing a personal shorthand in addition to the sanctioned version, and fling our signatures across such an overwhelming volume of paperwork each day that style falls by the wayside. In particular, physician prescriptions for physical therapy are frequently written with such a dash and flair that you practically need a Rosetta stone to decipher the order. Perhaps due to my own poor calligraphic skills, I have an inherent talent for translating badly written orders.

Lauren backed out of the room, smiling and nodding to her new patient within while holding up her left hand in the universal gesture meaning "just wait a moment and I'll be right back." She raced back to the small room where we did our daily charting, and spied me industriously scrawling the day's findings into my stack of patient charts. Perplexed, she said, "Check out this Rx—I can't read what it says, can you?" I took the paper from her, noting her confusion.

"What's going on?" I asked.

"Well, a really nice guy, thirty-nine years old, levator tear, started telling me his history, and it just kept getting weirder and weirder! He said his pain worsened with sitting, and that he also had trouble walking quickly . . . I kept trying to find out why this would have any effect whatsoever on his neck and shoulder, but he insisted on talking to me about uncomfortable chairs. Then, he confided that he could no longer ride his bicycle without excruciating pain in his butt, and could I look at it?! Do you just think he's being fresh with me, or what?"

I looked closely at the prescription, and started to laugh. "Lauren, it says here he has a levator ani tear, not a levator scapulae tear! It *is* his butt! So, how do you plan to treat this?" Poor Lauren flushed red, and then set her jaw. "There's no way I can treat that diagnosis here. I'll have to tell him he's in the wrong sort of clinic . . . outpatient orthopedics just isn't the right place for a rectal problem, no matter how the injury occurred!"

Part Three

The Upper Extremities

A brave arm makes a short sword long.
—Author unknown

The components of the upper extremities are meant to work seamlessly together to give us the ability to reach, lift, push, pull, and throw our arms around one another in an embrace. There is a necessary balance between the work of the larger muscles that provide stability to the shoulder blade and the smaller muscles surrounding the shoulder joint, elbow, wrist, hand, and fingers, which allow fine movements such as those that we use when signing our names. Perhaps the stiffness in my own shoulder and elbow joints, born from bending over a multitude of patients throughout the years, has contributed to the scrawling quality of my signature. My husband teases me that all the women in my family write in the same cramped, spiky manner, and that he can read none of our secret missives to each other—all he can make out are the two "A's" that begin the first and last names of my signature. Nonetheless, the same hand that dents the page with my firm cursive is also able to caress, soothe, and perform delicate forms of treatment on the ailing bodies of family, friends, famous athletes, secret government agents, and ordinary people.

Gray Hair Means Cuff Tear

I ask not for a lighter burden, but for broader shoulders.
—Jewish proverb

The shoulder complex is one of the greatest wonders of the human body both physically and spiritually. We face the world shoulder-to-shoulder in solidarity, offer our shoulders for each other to cry or lean on, clap our friends on the back in encouragement, pat our loved ones on the shoulder to comfort them, and resolutely "shoulder our burdens" when necessary. Despite its temperamental nature, the shoulder is one of my favorite parts of the body to treat because it is highly responsive to therapeutic intervention. When we can visualize and understand the intricate interconnection of the associated muscles, tendons, ligaments, bones, and connective tissues, we can begin to properly approach this complicated body part. Since the glenohumeral joint is the most freely moving joint in the body, it is also extremely vulnerable to injury, offering interested therapists frequent opportunities to practice our skills.

The shoulder girdle consists of the clavicle, scapula, and glenohumeral joint. The only true bony link between the shoulder girdle and the rest of the skeleton is the small sternoclavicular joint where the clavicle, or collar bone, inserts into the sternum. All other parts of the shoulder complex are freely floating, controlled effortlessly by the coordinated contraction and relaxation of our shoulder, chest, and back muscles. Every arm motion begins with a stable scapula, which is held in position against the rib cage by a sling of strong muscle attachments. From this position of scapular stability the glenohumeral joint is able to coordinate its freedom via the rotator cuff muscles, in a pattern known as "mobility on stability."

Whenever we lift an arm, the scapula must perform a controlled slide across the ribcage, using strength and leverage, like a rock climber belaying a more nimble companion safely across a rock face, to allow the glenohumeral joint constrained yet uninhibited movement. The entire complex is fine-tuned by the nerves that originate in the cervical spine and flow down the arm via the brachial plexus nestled within the axilla. None of the muscles will work properly without the energizing flow of action potentials through the network of nerves that "tell" the muscle fibers when and how to contract.

~ ★ ~

Jeff strode up to me purposefully as he entered the office, pushing the clinic door open with his left hand with such force that it hit the back wall with a resounding crack. I reached out to shake his hand, and was puzzled to discover that he had to literally throw his right hand into mine before being able to grasp my hand to shake it. Jeff's prescription read "Shoulder and Back Pain," shedding scant light upon his actual problem.

"I'm very active," Jeff said confidently. "I go to yoga twice a week, work out in aerobic and weight training, and try hard to stay fit. But a few weeks ago, I had some right shoulder pain that came down into my hand on a business trip, and when I got home again the pain went away, but I started to notice that my shoulder blade was sticking into the seat behind me when I lifted my arms onto the steering wheel to drive. It's making me crazy!"

"What does your doctor think is going on?" I asked.

"He thinks I strained something in my shoulder, so he sent me here."

As usual, the climate control system in the clinic was misbehaving. It was accustomed to spewing forth heat in the summer and air conditioning in the winter to an accompaniment of clicking and banging noises. Consequently, I never knew how to dress when going to work, as the system would fluctuate wildly according to its own whims. On this chilly late October morning the air conditioning kicked on with a grunt, at odds with the turtleneck I was wearing beneath my lab coat. I apologized to Jeff about the frigid conditions, but insisted that in order to see his shoulder and back properly, I would need to have him lift his shirt up. "No problem," he responded, dragging off his long-sleeved shirt awkwardly as he turned his back to me.

In that one faltering moment, I saw the cause of his problem—his right scapula was winging away from his ribcage, unable to stabilize his glenohumeral joint enough to control the necessary arm elevation as he tried to manipulate the long-sleeved shirt over his head. "Oh no," I blurted, "I think you might have a nerve injury."

Jeff spun around, saying, "What do you mean? The doctor said I probably just strained the muscles around my shoulder blade, which makes them feel swollen and as if they're sticking out more."

"To some extent that's true, since the uninjured muscles now have to work extra hard to try to control your shoulder blade, but unfortunately the reason your scapula is sticking out is that the nerve 'feeding' the muscles that coordinate its movement is asleep," I said. "It's a classic case—somewhere along the path of the nerve, maybe the long thoracic nerve, there is an area where it's being compressed or a place where it got overstretched. Can you remember anything about your business trip that might have compressed your arm? Did you get involved in a meeting where you were turned toward someone in conversation, your right arm draped over the back of your chair? Or, did you get drunk and fall asleep with your arm in an awkward position?" I asked with a small smile. "This type of nerve injury is also known as 'Saturday night palsy' due to the vulnerability of the nerve to compressive forces—if its owner passes out and inadvertently sleeps on the arm for a prolonged period of time, that can trigger the injury. Or, were you dragging luggage around behind you on its wheels? That might have tractioned the nerve, causing a stretch injury."

Jeff smiled ruefully, "Nothing nearly as exciting as a drunken binge on this trip; but, I wonder if the luggage pulling, or maybe the battle of the overhead bin on the airplane, was a problem."

Unfortunately, the average rate of peripheral nerve regeneration is thought to be about one millimeter per day, and during the healing process little can be done other than to carefully exercise the unaffected muscles surrounding the denervated ones, to maintain joint health with a daily range of motion regimen for all of the joints in the affected extremity, and to then gradually rebuild strength in the sleepy muscles as the nerve messages are slowly restored.

It is frustrating for these patients to have to simply wait it out. I taught Jeff a home exercise program to stretch out his tight pectoral and anterior deltoid muscles, strengthen the support muscles around his scapula, and exercise everything else in the area until his serratus anterior muscle chose to reawaken, like Sleeping Beauty. In cases such as Jeff's, the affected area can take up to a year and a half to regain normal function. After arming Jeff with information and a progression of exercises, we settled down to wait.

~ ★ ~

One of the reasons I eventually decided to return to outpatient orthopedic physical therapy, after trying home health, acute rehab, neuro rehab, hippotherapy, and geriatric rehab, was the desire to improve my skills with the ordinary problems that my loved ones came up against the most frequently. Some of my PT friends had stars in their eyes, hoping to rub shoulders with famous athletes, but I simply wanted to be able to help my family and friends with their everyday, nonglamorous injuries and restore both their physical comfort and their peace of mind. I have treated Olympic athletes, CIA agents, and well-known sports figures, but my heart always gravitates toward "ordinary" people. When Granny was ninety years old and still living independently in her flat in the north of England, she was burglarized. As the thief exited, he pushed her down the stairs in his haste, breaking her shoulder in the process. Because of her advanced age, Granny's rehabilitation was difficult. Her shoulder "froze" as it recovered, and she needed physical therapy to recover her flexibility and strength so that she could once again independently put on her bras, vests, and sweaters. I saw how much the therapy affected her ability to be able to live alone again, and I wanted to be able to help someone else's grandmother in the same way.

Each part of the body has its own characteristics and moods, and responds differently to therapeutic intervention. This corporeal tendency reminds me of the old horseman's adage of how to deal with recalcitrant horseflesh: "You ask a mare, tell a gelding, and consult with a stallion." The uniquely individual responses seen in the personalities of the horse world are reflected in the human body. In my experience, shoulders are temperamental, knees are stoic, and elbows are grumpy. The shoulder takes the light touch and sensitive hand of a caring therapist to be guided back to wellness, as the rotator cuff is so easily damaged by many seemingly benign therapeutic techniques.

During the early years of practice, this sensitive feel takes some time and experience to develop. Countless patients are unknowingly injured as neophyte PTs attempt to stretch out their patient's shoulder stiffness by inadvertently jamming the supraspinatus and long head of the biceps tendons beneath the acromial arch of the shoulder blade. This is especially easy to do in the patient with a frozen shoulder, also known as adhesive capsulitis. With adhesive capsulitis, the glenohumeral joint capsule becomes inflamed and stiffens, or "freezes" into a tightened position that severely restricts the movement of the entire arm. Even at rest, the shoulder feels like it is being attacked by breathtakingly sharp bolts of lightning, and any attempted movement makes it scream in agony.

~ ★ ~

"My doctor says I have 'fifties shoulder,'" June explained grimly in disgusted tones. "What did I do to deserve this? There has been no accident, no injury, no reason for it! It constantly hurts, and stabs at me if I move too quickly . . . and forget trying to fasten my bra or get comfortable in bed at night. Besides, I'm only forty-two years old!"

I squinted at June's prescription, which read "Adhesive Capsulitis—Evaluate and Treat." In Chinese cultures this condition is also known as fifties shoulder, since it commonly occurs between the ages of forty and sixty-five. Adhesive capsulitis can be classified as primary or secondary, with primary adhesive capsulitis spontaneously occurring from an unknown stimulus and secondary adhesive capsulitis manifesting in response to prior trauma, degenerative changes in the shoulder joint, or from disuse of the arm from immobilization in a sling after traumatic injury. Adhesive capsulitis has been associated with underlying medical conditions such as diabetes and rheumatoid arthritis, and is more frequently seen in women than men, although in many cases the underlying pathology remains frustratingly hidden. Anecdotally, I have noticed many adhesive capsulitis cases occurring at times of life changes, such as moving to a different state, retiring, going through menopause, experiencing the death of a loved one, or trying to complete a doctoral thesis. Fortunately, it is more likely to crop up in the nondominant rather than the dominant shoulder.

Despite being somewhat young for the typical patient with adhesive capsulitis, June fit the profile in other ways. She was in the information-gathering stage of writing her doctoral thesis in psychology and had been experiencing the accompanying stresses of lack of sleep and declining interpersonal interactions under a looming deadline, in addition to laboring under the label of being premenopausal. June had suffered through the initial "freezing" phase of the adhesive capsulitis, during which time her left shoulder had become acutely inflamed and had progressively stiffened up, and was now in the midst of the "frozen" phase. The extreme stiffness and pain of her shoulder was severely limiting her ability to sleep, concentrate, and even use the computer to work on her thesis. Some researchers feel that the diagnosis of adhesive capsulitis is a self-limiting one and that given enough time the shoulder will "thaw" on its own. However, most health professionals agree that even if this is true, physical therapy treatment to assist the limbering up process is desirable to reduce pain and to speed up the recovery phase.

June looked at me crankily, challenging me to suggest that she looked closer to thirty than fifty years old. In truth, after many late nights working on her manuscript, she definitely looked her age. Her pale skin was lined, there were dark circles etched beneath her eyes, and her fair, flyaway hair was untended. She took a swig of white liquid from her water bottle and said, "I'm so dry! The doctor wanted me to take painkillers before coming in here, since it's supposed to be so painful during the therapy."

"What is that you're drinking?" I asked curiously.

"Milk! I love it, and drink it all the time. This is my second bottle of the day," June replied.

I said, "Better you than me—I haven't been able to drink milk since I was seven years old."

June looked at me curiously, her prickliness dissipating. "Why not?" she asked. "Are you lactose intolerant?"

"Well no, it's actually my Dad's fault," I answered. "I grew up in an airline family, and we traveled all over the place all the time . . . on a trip to South Africa, we had to take anti-malaria pills as a precaution, but I hated the taste because they were really bitter. I would hide the pill under my tongue and then run outside and spit it out behind the hut where we were staying. After my parents discovered my little evasion, I was made to take the pill in front of them and wash it down with milk. The problem was, the milk was rubbery and thick, and my Dad joked that it was impala milk and not from a cow at all! I just couldn't make myself drink milk anymore after that." June chuckled, and took another swig of milk.

I asked, "What is the subject of your thesis?" as I began to gently assess her shoulder range of motion. Her expression softened as she responded, "How music subconsciously affects the psyche. Have you ever had the experience of hearing a song in your mind, usually an older song from your past, and then realized that it was making you feel a particular emotion during a certain time?"

I nodded in agreement as I carefully stretched her upper arm away from her rib cage and measured her available abduction. "Do you mean, like when I'm feeling irritated at a rude sales clerk and then realize the lyrics playing in my head are 'I'm going to tell that girl to shut up, I'm going to tell that girl I'm going to beat her up'?" I joked.

"Yes, that's it exactly!" June said. "I'm doing a study in which I'm asking people to pay attention to the song-in-the-head phenomenon and write down (a) which song it is, (b) what emotions they were feeling at the time they realized they were mentally replaying the song, and (c) what the situation was. The ultimate goal will be to use songs and lyrics in a positive way, and to have people actively influence their emotions by consciously and purposefully remembering certain songs to make themselves feel better."

June flinched as I moved her arm passively into external rotation. Forty-five degrees—she was extremely tight. Most people are able to cock their arms back into the pitching position to at least 90 degrees, but June's glenohumeral joint capsule had tightened down so much, it was as if she was trying to wring out a short, shrunken washcloth. "Sorry," I murmured as I slowly released her arm. "Your study sounds really interesting, and I have actually noticed that phenomenon before with emotionally laden bits of music . . . if you're still looking for study participants once I've helped you with your shoulder problem and you're no longer my patient—conflict of interest, you know—I'd like to help! In the meantime, let's measure how flexible your right shoulder is so we can see how far off this left one actually is."

After examining June's active and passive range of motion, strength, reflexes, and muscle tone, we discussed her functional limitations. Then, I cradled her shoulder cautiously in my hands and lightly felt for the limits of glenohumeral joint excursion and for the end-feel, or the quality of resistance I could detect through my hands at the farthest reaches of the joint's accessory motion (the ability of the joint to glide, spin, and roll in order to achieve volitional movement). June had significantly restricted anterior-posterior glide as well as nearly nonexistent inferior glide of the ball within the socket. Her end-feel was painful from her perspective, and firm and rubbery (capsular) from mine. She had a classic primary adhesive capsulitis. "The doctor wants to do a manipulation on my shoulder," June volunteered, "but the whole thought of being put under and then having the doctor crack my shoulder apart scares me! I'm really hoping that the PT can do the job instead."

I began treating her shoulder with gentle, oscillatory gliding mobilizations of the glenohumeral joint to reduce her pain and to gingerly extend the available joint range of motion. Without restoration of the joint's gliding accessory movements, physiologic motion is blocked—in other words, if the ball cannot slide a little within the socket to reach and maintain a central position, normal arm movement becomes restricted. "What song do you have playing in your head right now?" I enquired as I carefully stretched her shoulder into a fresh position and she sighed.

"That Nina Gordon song," June replied in surprise. "You know, the one with the lyrics that go 'Down to the earth I fell with dripping wings, heavy things won't fly'—but you know, I love that song and it seems so hopeful when the lyrics go on to say 'Gleaming in the dark sea I'm as light as air, floating there breathlessly . . . I feel so light, this is all I want to feel tonight'—ha! That's promising . . ." she said thoughtfully. Then, she suddenly said, "I need to sit up; I'm feeling a little lightheaded." Her shoulder suddenly felt clammy beneath my hands, and I knew what that meant. I quickly sat her up, and raced for the garbage can. In the nick of time, I whipped the can in front of her as she vomited up what seemed like gallons of sour-smelling impala milk. The painkillers had won the battle over June's stomach lining, despite the milk coating.

Over a series of our sessions together I continued focusing on gentle, repeated mobilization of the glenohumeral joint with rhythmic, oscillating inferior and anterior-posterior glides. As if in slow motion, June's shoulder unfurled like a blooming springtime flower, and as it did, the pain faded away and she was able to begin to use the arm again to tuck in her shirt, pull up the bedclothes, and lift up her laptop computer. Eventually, the long-awaited day arrived when June was able to fasten her bra behind her back. She said, "I have to go and see the doctor again for a recheck to see if I still need the manipulation, but I hope not—what do you think?"

"I think that you're doing so well now I'd be surprised if Dr. M would want to do a manipulation," I responded. "You've come one heck of a long way, and frankly your range of motion is too good for a manipulation! In fact, I know he's really pleased with your progress because I sent him a report yesterday and he's already faxed his response back to me—look, you can see his comment right here," I said as I held the signed prescription out to her. The doctor had sent back an updated prescription requesting that I continue working with June for another month, and had added "Excellent progress!!!"

When I next saw June, she had just returned from her recheck appointment with the doctor. Smiling, she handed me a paper and said, "You promised."

"What's this?" I asked.

"Your consent form for my thesis. I'm doing so much better now that I think you'll be able to participate in my study as we finish our time together since we're on the home stretch! I want you to track your thoughts each day, and hone in on three major episodes in which you notice a correlation between the songs in your head, the situations you're in when you become aware of the songs, and your emotional state during those times," she responded. "Don't be surprised if the songs that are triggered are older ones that link to events in your past; but, at the same time, there is no right or wrong answer. Just relax and have fun with it!"

Ah. I did promise, didn't I? And so, I found myself embarking upon a journey of self-discovery. The first day, my brain remained unusually and stubbornly quiet. Perhaps I was no good at this psychological thing, and besides, I had never been particularly musical. But I was intrigued by the possibilities. Could my unconscious emotional state be brought to light through remembered song lyrics? Was this a window into my inner psyche? Would consciously thinking about it too much influence the outcome? It seemed like a form of dream therapy. I did a little research on music therapy and discovered that when individualized forms of music are played during surgery, therapy sessions, or even in the patient's hospital room, people felt better and doctors report that the recovery is faster. I had long been aware that patients with Parkinson's disease were able to unlock their rigid, shaking bodies more easily in the presence of music, which seemed to facilitate their ability to walk with longer, easier strides. I had also learned of a theory that patients with Alzheimer's disease would become less agitated and sleep better in the presence of meaningful or calming music. These studies of passive music listening seemed to aptly describe the soothing, healing qualities of sound, but failed to address the potential for remembered songs to examine the psyche, or to examine the reverse—if songs were a window of the inner emotions, could one conversely heal emotional pain with the deliberate selection of certain songs? I decided to clear my mind and see what happened.

Later that day, I mentioned the thesis project to another patient, Freddie, who was a nurse in the local hospital's intensive care unit as well as a friend. She said, "Oh, sure, that happens all the time. When I was in labor with my son in the 1960s, the song 'Chains of Love' played over and over in my head; I just couldn't get rid of it!" I joked, "Did that turn out to be symbolic of the relationship you have with your son?"

"Yes," she replied shortly.

There were a few false starts. When I hurriedly left work to go visit my horse before darkness fell, I heard two seagulls mewing overhead as I walked to my car. Almost immediately, the song "I Ran (So Far Away)" by none other than the group A Flock of Seagulls began to play in my head—I suppose at least my unconscious mind had a sense of humor.

With my mind's ear newly cupped in the direction of my subconscious mind, songs began to rattle through my head fast and furiously. Over the following weeks, I noticed that during times of stress lyrics from the song "Living on a Thin Line," recorded by the old British band The Kinks, would waft into my consciousness.

But I wasn't merely content to let the music take over and fill my seemingly passive brain. I started to actively employ music to try to change my mood, focusing on thinking about happy or soothing tunes when I was anxious or agitated. In the beginning, I found that this was only marginally effective. Perhaps because I am such a visually oriented person, internal auditory cues do not have the power to easily change my state of mind. I am quite sure that research is ongoing, but I derive a much greater benefit from imagining visual images. I usually have trouble falling asleep at night regardless of my level of fatigue, and I toss and turn for many half-hour segments until I slump into exhausted sleep. My husband always tells me to imagine looking at a blank wall to quell my darting thoughts, but this method is too passive for me and I cover the wall with the graffiti of my feelings. Instead, late at night as I lie tensely with whirling thoughts and images pounding my brain, I imagine taking a huge cooking spatula in my right hand. Armed with this mental tool, I then steadily dip the spatula into a large vat of creamy vanilla cake frosting and repeatedly smooth the contents directly onto a sheet of clear plate glass that is suspended in front of the scenes playing through my brain. Usually, by the time I've completely frosted the scene over, I am deep in refreshing slumber.

On nights when my subconscious mind focuses too much on trying to eat the frosting, I will mentally walk through my grandmother's Victorian home on Diamond Street in North Yorkshire, a place I haven't been inside for more than twenty years. I figuratively hang up my childhood red anorak in the hall where I greet the oil painting of an ancestor (which is reputed to fall down off the wall whenever a family member is about to die), peek into the front room to visit with my grandfather, and make my way into the scullery to bake a coffee cake with Granny. Then, I continue my tour of the house, greeting happy memories and family heirlooms and stroking the spines of favorite books, and by the time I reach the box room in the attic I am asleep, with a nostalgic smile on my face.

In the slow hours of the night I can most easily fall into a dreamlike state by mentally summoning these visual images, perhaps because although my dreams are rich in visual and somatic detail, they are usually silent. But during the busy daytime hours I was eventually able to teach myself to actively select songs that had the power to lift my spirits or make me laugh. Before long, I became skilled at employing both visual and auditory imagery to ease not only my anxieties but also those of my patients. During treatment, it is especially helpful to take patients on guided visualizations of happy times or encourage them to recall significant, comforting songs to lull them into a relaxed frame of mind as I aggressively mobilize and stretch a stiff shoulder bound down by adhesions.

~ ★ ~

Over the years I have developed a bit of a knack for treating the temperamental shoulder, and like most therapists am able to hone my perceptive touch to the extent that I can sense minute increases in the joint's resistance as I mobilize the joint into end range. This enhanced feel allows me to sense where the joint's lim-its are and to modify my mobilization techniques to stretch tight joint capsules and stiff glenohumeral joints in a delicate dance. My husband teases me that I am the "best therapist in the Tri-Valley area," a source of amusement since the part of the Bay Area where we live contains only a single valley. One of the greatest fac-tors in developing my sense of feel has been the ongoing battle with my own shoulder stiffness.

Over the years, I had noticed an increasing tendency for my right shoulder to succumb to impingement syndrome, in which the supraspinatus and long head of the biceps tendons would become trapped beneath my acromion with certain movements. It was a struggle to keep the shoulder comfortable when I reached out to demonstrate exercises or massage and mobilize my patients' injured bodies. Although my shoulder pain remained manageable for a long time, I eventually began to perceive trouble in the bedroom. I would feel sharp little needles stick-ing into my shoulder when flicking the duvet straight in the mornings as I made the bed, and was unable to lie on my right shoulder without my entire arm, hand, and fingers becoming numb. As a typical health professional, I was slow to seek help for myself and simply soldiered on by compensating more with my left arm and by avoiding my right side during the night.

Then, one day a colleague and I were leaning against the wall chatting as we waited for our next patients to arrive. Jill was engrossed in a story about one of her patients with poor posture and shoulder problems and casually said, "He looks a lot like you, you know . . . in fact, I'll bet your shoulders are even stiffer than his!"

Rising to the challenge, I immediately made Jill measure my shoulder active range of motion right there in the hallway. "No way," I asserted. "There's no way

I'm as stiff as your patient—I've seen him! Go ahead, measure my good side and I'll prove it," I said as I lifted my left arm into flexion, confidently reaching as far above my head as I could.

Measurements of normal shoulder range of motion in the position of forward flexion vary. Teenagers, young adults, and flexible older people who may have done yoga will show measurements anywhere from 165 degrees to 180 degrees, zero degrees being the position in which the arm is resting quietly at the side. But, we tend to get a bit stiffer as we age, so older people and those over age sixty-five are more likely to have a measurement of 150 degrees to 165 degrees. Jill lined the goniometer up against my left arm and rib cage, and reported, "148 degrees." I was stunned. This was my flexible, pain-free shoulder! In a panic, I cried, "You're kidding! Measure the right one, quick." Jill obediently shifted over to the other side and measured my right arm as I forced it overhead with a wince. After a moment, she declared, "135 degrees." Oh my. No wonder it was giving me such trouble; the joint was severely restricted for someone my age and was squeezing my rotator cuff tendons between the acromion and the head of the humerus with practically every movement. It was time for the therapist to try to heal herself.

I soon found that it is impossible to mobilize one's own shoulder joint. So, I enlisted the help of my husband after I asked another colleague to properly assess my painful right shoulder. He discovered that my humeral head had anteriorly subluxed and that I had virtually no inferior glide. Although my shoulder wasn't frozen (internal and external rotation were nearly normal), it was, as they say, bloody tight. There is an old adage in the therapy world, "Gray hair means cuff tear," so I was motivated to reduce my shoulder stiffness in order to decrease the risk of fraying my rotator cuff tendons as they rubbed against the bone. It was, and still is, an ongoing struggle.

~ ★ ~

Most of us will face some degenerative changes somewhere in our bodies as we get older, the only mystery being which part will start to go wrong. The shoulders, bearers of our burdens and responsibilities, are a common target for pain. Shoulder arthritis and degenerative joint disease are often associated with a family history of osteoarthritis, previous injury to the joint, and aging.

As degenerative changes occur, the joint space between the acromion and the humeral head becomes increasingly narrow, which can lead to impingement of the rotator cuff tendons as they become squeezed between the bones during upper extremity movement. Impingement syndrome can be caused by any condition that narrows the space between the humeral head and acromion, including normal anatomic variation that results in a downward-curving acromion, a thickened or calcified coracoacromial ligament, acromioclavicular (AC) joint arthritis, or underlying pathology in the rotator cuff that allows the humeral head to glide upward in the socket. Impingement can also be caused by the formation of bone spurs (osteophytes), which hang down into the joint space like little cave stalactites, digging into the underlying tendons. Through my own battles with shoulder problems, I developed a fresh appreciation for the pain and stiffness of my fellow sufferers. So, when my husband said he had noticed that one of our friends was being tortured in the hot flames of shoulder hell, I leapt into the fray to offer my assistance.

"It hurts when I do this," said George as he raised his right upper arm and elbow above shoulder height in the classic chicken dance pose.

"Then don't do that," I cracked. "But seriously, don't raise your arm like that—with the shoulder in a position of internal rotation, you're putting your shoulder into a position where the tendons are easily squeezed and pinched between the bones . . . try to always raise your arm with the palm or the thumb pointing upward to help clear the tendons. Now, what other things make the pain worse?"

George replied, "Well, pretty much everything. The shoulder feels really stiff in general, but it's worse when I reach for things, when I lift and carry heavy buckets of sand, and after I work out in the gym. Lately, it's really been bothering me when I ride my motorcycle, maybe something to do with having to hold the throttle open with my arm raised in a tense position, and I have the hardest time shrugging out of my leathers after a ride! It's getting embarrassing, and I don't want to do anything girly like ask one of the other guys to help me."

I snorted and proceeded to assess George's shoulder, finding that he had terrible active range of motion in both shoulders after a lifetime of working in and then owning his own tile-setting business. The strain of mixing and lifting heavy buckets of wet sand for grout, combined with repeated overhead work setting innumerable tiles into his client's walls, was a recipe for shoulder arthritis and impingement. To compensate for his restricted glenohumeral joint when lifting the arm, George inadvertently shrugged his shoulder girdle into a hunched position in an effort to increase the span of his reach. Unfortunately, the shoulder hunching maneuver only serves to lift the scapula a few degrees, and can often result in neck and upper trapezius soreness. I asked, "Do you have any neck pain?"

"Yes, my neck can be pretty stiff and sore on the right side," he replied in surprise as he twisted his neck around. I observed that he was much more restricted into right cervical rotation, a pattern that fits with right upper trapezius pain and tightness.

George's neural tension was normal, and he had no signs of upper extremity numbness or tingling. His static resisted tests, in which the muscles and tendons are isometrically resisted to assess their strength and pain response, highlighted mild weakness and pain in the supraspinatus and biceps muscles. However, his passive joint range of motion was even more revealing. The right shoulder was markedly worse than the left, exhibiting a capsular pattern of tightness in the joint. When I carefully moved his arm into end range shoulder flexion, he winced and reported a sharp, pinching pain that radiated into his deltoid, a common spot for referred pain. With palpation of his shoulder structures, I found thickened "speed bumps" at the long head of the biceps tendon and at the insertion of the supraspinatus tendon. These bumpy, tender areas of increased soft tissue density were indicators of inflamed and thickened tendons. "Is this where you feel the most soreness?" I asked as I circumspectly pressed on the dense spots. George writhed in discomfort, saying, "Ouch! Hey—how do you know? Do you feel something there?" as I felt his sore tendons and told him about my findings.

The three of us concocted a plan—George would come over once a week after dinner armed with beer and dessert to chat about life, fast engines, and music with my husband (he and George were both avid motorcycle enthusiasts and guitarists), and then I would work on George's shoulder. After our sessions of joint mobilization, stretching, exercise instruction, and massage, we would take a break. Although I avoided the beer in the interest of professionalism, I enjoyed sampling my way through George's dessert picks—he very kindly focused on chocolate-based desserts to accommodate my preference.

We made a padded treatment table for him using the cats' purple blanket folded on top of our tile kitchen counter so that I could mobilize his shoulder without kneeling over him on the living room floor—the kitchen counter was nearly the perfect height for me to deliver accurate mobilizing pressures to his shoulder. In the beginning, George accented his pre-therapy beer with a shot or two of well-chilled vodka before building up his courage to let me work on him. However, as his shoulder loosened and he got used to my treatment techniques,

George became braver and simply relaxed with his beer and a chat with my husband before succumbing to my tender ministrations.

Between the adhesive capsulitis and the tendonitis, George's shoulder was a bit of a mess. He had the tendency to produce extra bone, as evidenced by his lumbar spinal stenosis, a condition in which additional bone forms around the spinal nerve roots and sometimes the spinal cord as well, positionally compressing the nerves into the legs. In light of his bone-producing tendencies and personal work history, I could only imagine that George might have developed superfluous bone on the underside of the acromion. I warned him that I would try to open up the restricted space between the humeral head and the acromion as best as I could, but there was always a chance that any large bone spurs might eventually have to be surgically removed.

Fortunately, as the weeks went by George responded slowly but surely with his shoulder movement and also his confidence. The three of us debated politics, engine power, and relationships. George was a paradox for the women he met, demonstrating Sir Galahad tendencies with the desire to rescue damsels in distress on the one hand, but a predisposition for Lone Wolf self-preservation on the other. Consequently, he would reel women in with his good-natured approachability and then back off as they became "too" interested. When the damsel perceived she was on the verge of losing him, she would go into hot pursuit and inadvertently chase him away. Conversely, the more aloof the women were, the more he was drawn in, becoming the pursuer in turn—George thrived on drama.

In Louise Hay's handbook *Heal Your Body*, the shoulders are said to represent our ability to carry life experiences joyously, with dysfunction in the shoulder region signifying an attitude of burden. Furthermore, the joints are thought to symbolize the ease with which we change direction in our lives. These concepts were interesting to consider, for as I made headway with George's sore right shoulder and he became more consistently pain free, he was successfully able to return to the dating scene after a long hiatus. More importantly, he was able to ride his motorcycle again without pain, which provided him with much-needed mental decompression.

~ ★ ~

At first I thought Josephine was just a crabby old woman. At five foot ten and seventy-five years of age, she had towered above most of her sisters and absorbed decades of wisdom and life experience. However, she often chose to look down at life with thinly veiled annoyance rather than to smile benignly upon it. Josephine's movements were very slow and measured, and despite the fact that she was invariably late for each therapy appointment, she never apologized for her tardiness or tried to quicken her stride. I quickly learned that if I leapt up from my sentry tower at the front desk, where I was catching up on my chart notes, and tried to hurry her along, she would stop dead in her tracks to regale me with some tale of woe, delaying the start of treatment even longer. She never seemed to show any emotion other than frustration, and would endlessly recite her soft-spoken list of complaints with a deadpan expression. However, everyone has her own path to walk, and it didn't take me long to begin to understand the frustrating mystery that was Josephine.

She had torn one of her rotator cuff tendons in a fall at an art museum, when she had tripped over a small bench as she backed away from a painting to view it more clearly. In an effort to save herself, Josephine had reached out with her right arm to grab onto her husband's arm but ended up catching his coat sleeve awkwardly instead. Her failing grasp slipped, and the next contact she had was with the polished marble floor. Amazingly, despite significant osteoporosis, she managed not to fracture anything but instead tore her subscapularis tendon and ripped apart her upper lip, loosening her front teeth. She was the most self-conscious about her lip, which resembled a harelip during the early stages of healing, but her greatest problem was the right shoulder. The subscapularis muscle is a large part of the rotator cuff, and is tucked away like an oyster inside its shell on the inner surface of the scapula against the rib cage. Its purpose is to help control the position of the humeral head with arm elevation and to internally rotate the arm, enabling us to reach up and hug each other. From what I could observe, it was difficult to imagine the last time Josephine had either given or received a hug.

On our initial encounter, Josephine reluctantly harrumphed her way onto the treatment table after first quizzing me about how often we cleaned the equipment, laundered the pillow cases, and bleached the towels. After reassuring her as to our strict standards of cleanliness, I was able to begin carefully assessing her right shoulder passive range of motion. Anticipating yet another complaint, I lifted her mildly trembling arm with great care. Then, I knew. In its relaxed state, Josephine's arm was abnormally stiff and gave ground to my gentle lifting force in a series of small ratcheting hiccups that were characteristic of the classic cogwheel rigidity of a certain neurological brain disorder—Josephine had

Parkinson's disease. In its early stages, Parkinson's disease tends to affect only one limb, creating slowed movements, a resting tremor, and rigidity in that limb. Josephine had mentioned earlier that she felt she didn't sleep well and that she frequently felt tired and sometimes clumsy or uncoordinated, additional signs that coincide with the onset of Parkinson's disease.

Other pieces of the puzzle began to rapidly slide into place as I thought about Josephine's arm and the manner in which she had walked into the clinic. Her overall posture was stiffly flexed forward, her gait pattern was shuffling and exhibited decreased stride length with increased double-leg stance time, and she had no arm swing as she walked along; in essence, she looked as if someone had left her parking brake on. Also, her facial expression was flat and her tone of speech monotonic, regardless of how agitated her views about hygiene were.

Josephine's Parkinson's disease was centered in her injured right upper extremity, the resultant stiffness and rigidity possibly playing a part in her unlucky art museum fall. Cautiously, I asked Josephine if she had seen any other health professionals recently such as a neurologist or physiatrist. She slowly replied, "Oh, yes—I suppose I should tell you that my neurologist says that I have Parkinson's disease. He says it's really quite mild, but I am taking Sinemet for it . . . I haven't told any of my friends, because I don't want to be pitied and I don't want them to treat me any differently. Do you think that has anything to do with my shoulder?" I said, "Only in the sense that the Parkinson's seems to have centered in your right arm. We'll just have to be careful that while your rotator cuff tear is healing, the shoulder doesn't become too stiff and try to freeze. Also, depending on how much the Parkinson's is affecting this arm, it may slow down your recovery just a bit. Sometimes an accident can aggravate the Parkinson's disease and vice versa, especially when head trauma is a factor."

From that point forward, I treated Josephine matter-of-factly and never referred to her Parkinson's disease again unless she was the one to bring it into the conversation. Instead, we focused on her shoulder, and as her trust in me grew, she steadily unbent toward me. Because of the Parkinson's disease, Josephine was unable to show overt signs of emotion, but she communicated her feelings quite clearly in her soft monotone. Eventually, her lip healed and her teeth stabilized in her gums—long before the range of motion returned to her shoulder. The limb rigidity that often accompanies Parkinson's disease is caused by the simultaneous muscle contraction of the flexor and extensor muscles, which can "lock" the affected limb and also the trunk. The abnormal muscular activity doesn't allow for the opposing muscle groups to relax, and they remain in a state of constant contraction, leading to stiffness. This problem became a real stumbling block to her recovery, as the underlying muscle tone frequently blocked Josephine's ability to actively move the arm at odd times.

"My arm locks in the middle of the night if I get out of bed to use the bathroom," Josephine complained. "I usually have to get up at least once a night, but I've taken to lying there in bed as long as I can stand it, because I know by the time I try to get back up off the toilet, I can't use my arm! It's like it gets glued to my side, and it takes a long time to loosen it up. Sometimes I can't even get up from the toilet, and I have to call and call until my husband wakes up to come and help me . . . I hate this disease!"

"Have you tried unlocking the right arm by moving the left arm around? Sometimes, exercises that use patterned or exaggerated movements like big rhythmic arm swings can break up Parkinson's stiffness," I said. "I know it feels like the arm is freezing up, but it's usually the co-contraction of the arm muscles fighting against each other that makes the arm stop moving, so what freezes can be unfrozen pretty quickly. The other thing you could try is an alternative movement to break up the tone. People with a locked arm or leg sometimes have success with attempting a completely different action, like shrugging your shoulder, blinking a few times in succession, or even humming a tune. Or, you could try rotating your right hand as if you're turning a doorknob—the body likes rotation, and it might help to unlock you faster, especially in the dead of night!" I explained.

"You always have such good ideas!" Josephine said. "I'll try them tonight."

When Josephine returned for our next appointment, she was much happier. "I found that if I wiggled my right wrist around and put a small hand towel as a spacer underneath my armpit to keep it away from my body, the arm didn't lock up on me as badly in the middle of the night," she reported. "I feel so much better, and it's great having some sense of control again. Now the problem I'm having is during the day. I was trying to paint a card for my husband's birthday—I used to do a lot of artwork, you know—and I just couldn't make my right hand hold the little brush. It's so frustrating! And I've noticed my handwriting is getting small and messy."

"Well, you're not alone there; you should see my scrawl," I joked. "It looks like something out of the Civil War era. But seriously, the resting tremor and rigidity you have in that right arm might be affecting your fine motor coordination a little. Sometimes it can be easier when you make the gripping surface bigger—in other words, if you build up the shaft of your paintbrush the way people put spongy sleeves on their pens and pencils, it might be easier for you to grip the brush. The other thing you could try is to simply assist and stabilize the right arm by holding the right wrist in your left hand to support it while you try to paint," I suggested.

Josephine's eyes teared up, glistening in joy at the thought of being able to continue to paint. "I love you," she cried. "I've been so depressed at the thought of having to give up the things I like, and then get worse and more disabled; this makes me feel so much more hopeful. I was so frustrated last night that I slammed my fist on the kitchen table and scared my husband," she said as she feebly pressed her left hand onto the treatment bench in a parody of mock outrage. "This is why I don't want to tell my friends—I'm afraid I'll frighten them all away!"

Over our time together, we were able to progressively stretch out her tight, injured subscapularis muscle and restore functional, although imperfect mobility to her shoulder. The fact that the Parkinson's disease was predominant in the injured arm meant that our progress was slow, but over the months Josephine steadily was able to regain independence. "I can drive the car now on the neighborhood streets!" she would say, or "I started to draw with charcoals again." One day she arrived toting a little canvas bag, late as usual.

"I hear you like chocolate," she said with a twinkle in her eye. "I just wanted to thank you for all your extra advice and care." With a trembling right hand, she carefully extricated a box of See's chocolate soft centers and held them out to me. I was touched, and also pleased to see that her right shoulder had recovered well enough to manage to control the path of the one-pound box. "Let's do one more exercise for your shoulder, Josephine," I said. "See if you can lift your right arm up high enough to give me a hug." She did, and said, "I needed that!" As we stepped away from each other, smiling with mutual affection, Josephine became serious.

"Don't ever leave me!" she said. "I need your good common sense to help me through this. If you think that my shoulder has improved enough, can you help me with the Parkinson's? Or, could I just pay you to talk to for an hour once or twice a week? No one else in my family seems to understand."

My heart wrung in sympathy for her. I said, "Josephine, we're talking right now! Besides, you're a smart woman, and you make great decisions all on your own; you don't need me for that."

Josephine said, "But I do need you! My sister is too busy to help me, plus she lives five hundred miles away. My daughter is always trying to get us to move into a retirement place, and I'm just not ready; I love our home . . . but my husband gets frustrated with me because it takes me such a long time to do anything around the house, and he doesn't understand how tired I feel most of the time. You're like the voice of reason; you understand me and always have such good suggestions for ways I can function better. I'm scared when I think about the future . . . you're better than any psychologist."

I patted Josephine awkwardly on her shoulder, and reassured her, "Well I'm glad I can be helpful, but I'm no psychologist! I simply point out a few things from time to time that might be helpful, and I care about what happens to you."

"You're a Florence Nightingale to me," she responded as we made our way out into the gym to try a few more exercises together.

~ ★ ~

Physical therapists are frequently seen as confidants by their patients, perhaps due in part to the intimate nature of hands-on treatment. Putting my hands on some-one inevitably seems to open the floodgates of emotion. At times this can be uncomfortable, especially when it's time to treat a co-worker; in such situations, the lines between personal and professional relationships can become as blurred as ink on paper in the rain.

Victoria had been calling in sick on Mondays and Fridays with increasing fre-quency, leaving Jack and myself in the lurch again and again. Without the benefits of an aide to help us set up patients on heat or ice, answer phones, schedule appointments, do the laundry, and perform hundreds of other tasks in the small outpatient clinic, our treatments would become fragmented as we scampered from room to room on hyperdrive, apologies flowing like water. Then, one Sunday Victoria left a message on the clinic answering machine to say that she had seen an emergency room doctor that day and wouldn't be able to work for at least a week, "even though I can't afford to take the time off—but it's really bad, they gave me muscle relaxants and painkillers and I can hardly move." Jack and I looked askance at each other, wondering what it was this time: we had already run through vol-umes of Victoria's previous episodes of food poisoning, ear infection, influenza, vomiting, diarrhea, sinus infection, and vertigo. Grimly, Jack asked her to come in to the clinic anyway to see if there was anything we could do to help.

Victoria stumped angrily into the clinic with reddened eyes and a martyred expression, clutching a physician order in her shaking hand. "I could barely make the drive over. My neck's killing me, I can't move my right arm, and my hand and

fingers are all numb," she said grumpily. "I think it's carpal tunnel or something."
In a surly mood, Victoria took me aside and said, "I'm just so mad at Jack I could
spit nails! I shouldn't even be here, but should be lying down and taking my medication." I told her that since she was here anyway, maybe I could help take a look
at her and do something to diminish her pain. Grudgingly, she agreed.

Without moving her neck or right arm, Victoria slowly made her way to the
last available treatment room in the clinic, complaining, "Well it just figures that
the only room left is nasty old room four. I hate this room. It's so small and dark,
and all the other ones have windows—I feel like a second-class citizen stuck back
here." I settled her into a chair and started to ask about her pain pattern. Earlier
during the previous week she had complained about having right shoulder pain
that sounded like biceps tendonitis when reaching for the computer mouse or
patient co-payments at the front desk, but had refused to let me help her. This
time, I was able to get her to move her neck (normal range of motion with slight
stiffness into right rotation), right shoulder (reluctance to actively raise the arm
more than 90 degrees into flexion or abduction), elbow (within functional limits,
or WFL), wrist (WFL), hand (WFL), and fingers (WFL). Strength testing and
reflexes were normal, and she had no neural tension signs. Hmm. I asked, "Where
exactly do you feel the tingling?"

Victoria replied, "All over in my right wrist and hand."

"Which part of the wrist and hand?" I clarified. "Just certain fingers, or all of
them, or a certain part of the hand, or what?"

"The whole hand," she said.

"Good news, then," I enthused. "You don't have carpal tunnel syndrome! That
has a specific distribution of tingling and numbness, so that lets you out—whew,
what a relief!"

Victoria looked discomfited. Quickly, I had her lie on the treatment table
and asked her to relax so I could feel the available passive range of motion in her
right shoulder. Trembling as violently as a scared Chihuahua, Victoria let me hold
her right arm but wouldn't let it go. "Relax, relax—I promise I won't drop it," I
encouraged as I moved her shoulder. But it was impossible. There was an empty
end-feel, so named because she refused to allow her arm to move as freely as it
was physically able to. From my perspective, there was no natural buildup of
joint resistance that normally occurs at the end of the range, but instead Victoria
guardedly pulled her arm away from my coaxing pressure. Giving up for the
time being, I asked her to roll up her sleeve so I could palpate the structures of
the shoulder. Her right upper trapezius and pectoral muscles were a little tight.

Then, at last! A concrete finding—on Victoria's right biceps tendon lurked an extremely small area of increased soft tissue density and swelling. As I gently felt the tiny bump, Victoria almost leapt off the treatment table and squealed in pain. "That's it!" she exclaimed. "I normally have a really high tolerance for pain, but this is terrible . . . what is it? Do I have tear? Should I ask for an MRI? Will I need surgery?"

I struggled to control my features as I summoned up the reserves of my patience. After all, the bump on Victoria's mildly inflamed biceps tendon was minuscule compared to what Jack and I worked with every day, both with our patients and in our own bodies. Soothingly, I murmured that it was just a little tendonitis and should soon be better with some treatment. Chastened, Victoria conceded, "Well, this was bothering me last week but I didn't like to say anything. You guys come in here and work with much worse injuries—heck, you were even in here when you had pneumonia! I guess it could be a lot worse." I decided not to say anything.

As I worked on Victoria's shoulder with joint mobilization to reduce her mild impingement, stretching to loosen the tight support muscles, and gentle cross fiber friction massage and ultrasound to increase the circulation at the tiny spot of inflammation, she started confiding in me. She had been in a verbally abusive relationship for five years during which time she had supported her live-in significant other while he was unemployed. Rather than treat her with gratitude, he repaid her by escalating his abuse. Victoria said that this, combined with her battles with depression and subsequent weight gain, made her feel trapped and hopeless. Her burdens felt too great to shoulder anymore alone, and she herself needed a shoulder to lean on.

Fixing Victoria's shoulder was the easy part, but mending her life was not so simple. We drew up lists of options (pro, con) about what she might do, and I listened to her daily heartsick reflections about the unfairness of it all. Then one sunny Saturday, I returned from a peaceful trail ride on my horse, Atlas, to find a message on my answering machine. It was Jack. Apparently, Victoria had called him to say she wished us well but she was leaving town and wouldn't be coming in to work any more. She had found a way out from under all of her burdens, and was returning home to her sister in another state. Running away? Solving her problems? Simplifying her life? We couldn't judge her, as everyone has her own path to follow. In the end, we would never know what became of Victoria, other than to recognize that her tolerance for pain of any kind had hit rock bottom.

I recognize that my own shoulder pain ebbs and flows in a synchronized dance with my patients' progress. Whenever I am having a run of especially challenging or worrisome cases, my impingement worsens and disturbs my sleep and peace of mind. During the long, wakeful hours in the quiet of the night when my shoulder pain chases away sleep, I listen to my husband's even breaths and feel the comforting weight of our cats' warm furry bodies leaning in against my legs as I plan a new approach or strategy to help my patients toward wellness. Each pain I have personally experienced represents a lesson learned or a condition understood.

~ ★ ~

When we wake up each morning, there is usually no clue as to how the day will go. Frequently, days that I think will be stressful because of a full patient schedule and stacks of unwritten progress reports are smooth and trouble free, and conversely, days that present themselves as a let-up in the weekly scramble sometimes disintegrate into a free-for-all of anxiety and stress. Consequently, we generally never know when we are about to receive a gift of meeting a new, special person. In addition, even when we do meet someone who is to become a unique and meaningful friend, we may not recognize this right away. Of course, there are exceptions, and in my life, two people stand out.

The first time I remember meeting my aunt I was a willful, self-absorbed child of five. We were in Scotland for my aunt's wedding day, and I had the mumps. I remember being kept to the sidelines due to my lumpy, ungainly, fevered appearance, and amused myself by surreptitiously scavenging the guests' champagne glasses as soon as they set them down. I would quickly down the delicious fizz, and then resume my post at the edge of the room to enjoy the confusion and subsequent refilling of the drained glasses. At the time I had no idea how precious my future relationship with my aunt would become, but I recognized that champagne was to become my favorite drink. In later years, my aunt and uncle would watch my brother and I occasionally while my parents took a respite vacation; they reported being unable to get me to eat anything other than chocolate pudding for weeks on end. I must have been an extremely trying child.

Since we lived continents away from each other, I saw my aunt only on rare occasions until she passed through San Francisco on the way to a medical conference when I was in my late twenties. By then I had channeled my willfulness into motivation and had emerged from my lumpy introspective cocoon into a reasonably articulate, obliging butterfly. From the moment I saw my aunt from the perspective of my newly evolved state, I recognized a kindred spirit—we are now more like sisters or doppelgangers than aunt and niece, and the gift and depth of her relationship has brought me lasting happiness.

Most of my other significant friendships have evolved much more slowly, the only other exception being that with my husband. When I first met his gaze, a bolt of electricity ran through me, weakening my knees and lighting up my soul and I *knew*. We were married just over a year later.

When I met Freddie, no such immediate epiphany occurred. I was running late on one of those days that starts out deceptively simple but ends practically in tears as patients show up late or at the wrong time or on the wrong day altogether. My only thought was, great—a new evaluation to squeeze in at the end of the day when I'm running so far behind. As I pulled myself together at the front desk, I glanced at her prescription. "Two-Part Impacted Proximal Humerus Fracture—Evaluate and Treat." Wonderful. A nice, complicated way to end the day. At least this patient had been sent to me by my favorite doctor. Squaring my shoulders and plastering what I hoped was an encouraging smile onto my face, I headed for treatment room number four to meet her. When I opened the door, I was met by a statuesque blonde of indeterminable age (late forties? midfifties?) who was nursing her right arm in a sling. Succinctly, she gave me her history—intensive care unit nurse at the local hospital on the verge of retirement (late fifties?) who had been attending her nephew's wedding rehearsal dinner on a wet October night when she had fallen over a hidden step, breaking her shoulder in two places. The force of the fracture was at an awkward angle, which meant that she had impacted the bone of her right humerus such that it was now noticeably shorter than her left arm. Exhibiting the understated behavior typical of most health professionals, Freddie had realized that she had done "big damage" to her shoulder at the time of the fall but had refused to go to the local hospital until the next day so as not to spoil her nephew's special event. She told me that the treating physician had just rolled his eyes in mock despair when he looked at her X-rays and she admitted that the fall had taken place nearly twenty-four hours previously. Unfortunately, nothing could be done except to strap her right arm to her chest to keep it stable and quiet while it healed.

By the time I saw her, Freddie couldn't bathe or get dressed without the assistance of her significant other, couldn't reach for anything, and had definitely quit trying to wrestle with her bra. Because she had also severely sprained her left wrist during the fall, she was left without the use of either arm and wasn't even able to get herself on and off the toilet. Worst of all, she couldn't lift the arm to sweep her flaxen hair up into her characteristic ponytail. The shoulder was stiff, spectacularly swollen, and of course, constantly painful.

As I worked to help Freddie regain her flexibility, we came to know each other pretty well. Since she was a fellow health professional, Freddie had the no-nonsense, practical approach to healing that I did, and we struck a chord with each other as she painfully labored through her exercises according to schedule. Like me, Freddie had seen a lot and then some when it came to patient care, and shared my slightly dry, rather macabre sense of humor. It is always difficult to mentally leave your patients behind, and Freddie and I also shared the tendency to notice anomalies in our fellow humans even when "off duty." One day, Freddie described being at a nurses' get-together in the midst of a busy restaurant when she noticed one of her colleagues gazing raptly at a woman seated at an adjoining table. Freddie whispered, "What are you looking at?" as she followed her friend's stare. The other nurse whispered back, "Just check out those veins! I could get an eighteen-gauge needle in there, easy!" as they dissolved into gales of chortling merriment.

With my treatment and her diligence with the home exercise program, Freddie's shoulder slowly healed. Each time she revisited her orthopedic surgeon for a follow-up X-ray, I would send a progress report over with lists of her latest accomplishments in range of motion, strength, and functional ability. After her last visit to the physician, Freddie came back into the clinic and said, "What did you write in my progress note to the doctor? He was reading it in front of me, and at one point just burst into laughter." Bemused, I quickly scanned a copy of my note that I had retained in her chart, and slowly replied, "I think it's because of what I wrote under the category 'Functional Abilities'—I put in that now you are able to put your hair up into a ponytail independently."

Freddie laughed, "That must be it! I'm sure he thought that was pretty funny. I know it doesn't sound like that big a deal, but I don't feel like myself if I can't put my hair up."

"Well, just be glad that I didn't comment on your 'positive lipstick sign' in the report," I said.

"What's that?" she asked.

"You call yourself an ICU nurse, yet remain unaware of the highly important 'lipstick sign'?" I teased. "A 'positive lipstick sign' refers to the patient's state of mental health. Usually, for some time after injury or surgery we feel pretty crummy about ourselves and about life, and during those dark days when, for example, we can't put up our own hair or manage in the bathroom, we simply don't bother with extras. So, we're likely to be found morosely lying around in our sweatpants (if we can even pull 'em on!) with complete apathy toward our appearance, sometimes falling into a mild depression. Then, as we start to feel better and more like our normal selves, our interest in life is rekindled. When this happens, we start to feel brighter and resume our typical patterns of self-care, including dressing in colors other than black." Freddie grimaced in recognition—most of her therapy clothes were of the black family.

Freddie countered, "Even though I've been wearing a lot of black lately, I try to liven things up with a brightly colored overshirt or underwear to try to raise my spirits."

I said, "Yeah, I know just what you mean. In fact, all of my underwear is in slightly different shades of purple ranging from periwinkle to eggplant. I tell my husband, this way if I ever go missing, you'll be able to fill out the police report accurately by saying 'oh yes, my wife is five foot eight inches tall, with brown hair and light blue-gray eyes . . . and by the way, she was definitely wearing purple underwear today'!"

I went on, "I don't know if you're aware of this, but I've noticed that you haven't worn any lipstick until just two weeks ago . . . but now that your shoulder has started to behave itself, over the last few therapy visits you've been sporting a rather nice shade of pink! It's a sure sign that you're feeling better within yourself."

Elbows Are Grumpy

No man lives without jostling and being jostled; in all ways he has to elbow himself through the world, giving and receiving offence.
—*Thomas Carlyle, Scottish essayist and historian (1795–1881)*

The elbow acts as the body's club bouncer, functioning to look tough and to regulate how closely we allow our fellow human beings to get to us. The elbow provides essential leverage to the muscles that govern arm movement, and enables us to keep each other at arms' length or to draw each other close. The elbows are also eloquently expressive, making it possible for us to assess people's moods and receptivity through body language. By bending our elbows to fold our arms across our chests we can define personal space and ward off unwelcome advances of thought. We stick our elbows out as we navigate unfamiliar crowds, bristling like a porcupine extending its quills. When needing space around us to work, we require elbow room. Conversely, we can also "bend an elbow" to raise a glass as we socialize among friends. We use our elbows to nudge each other in laughter or to share a joke (nudge, nudge, wink, wink, à la Monty Python), and we rub elbows to hobnob with celebrities. When riding horses, we hold the reins by keeping a straight line from the elbow to the bit, and when joyously moving forward with friends, we link our arms at the elbows with them in solidarity.

But in addition to fine-tuning body language and helping with the heavy lifting, the elbow joint harbors a lesser-known secret. Although the elbow is famous for performing as a hinge joint, with the biceps and triceps muscles moving the ulna against the lower end of the humerus, it also enables the forearm to rotate. The simplest act of turning a doorknob or maneuvering a computer mouse is made possible only by the articulation of the forearm bones, known as the radius and the ulna, at the elbow. Although one of the most frequently seen diagnoses in outpatient orthopedic physical therapy clinics is that of tennis elbow, many other injuries can also occur at this seemingly sturdy site.

~ ★ ~

Lateral epicondylitis, or tennis elbow, is surprisingly common, usually affecting people during their active years between youth and middle age. Although most cases are caused by repetitive trauma that gradually results in microscopic tears and inflammation of the forearm tendons, it can also result from a single mis-guided movement. Because the elbow acts as a leverage point that connects the larger muscles of the trunk and shoulder to the smaller, more delicate muscles that control fine motor coordination, it is frequently placed under a great deal of stress.

When the forearm extensor tendons are strained, the injury is called tennis elbow, due to the high incidence of the condition in tennis players, who must perform resisted backhand strokes with an away-from-the-body movement. When medial epicondylitis occurs and the forearm flexor tendons are strained, the injury is called golfer's elbow, due to its high prevalence in golfers, who must forcefully drive the ball with an across-the-body motion. The vast majority of patients I see with either type of epicondylitis appear to obtain it without ever picking up a racquet or club; instead they tend to be repetitive computer mouse clickers, home do-it-yourselfers who repetitively twist their forearms, or those who must constantly grip or hold tools. On occasion, mousers who decide to pick up a new sport will come down with the dysfunction as well, in true "weekend warrior" fashion. However, many times the condition can be induced by trauma.

~ ★ ~

"I think I may have done something to my elbow," my husband said through clenched teeth as he made his way into the house from the garage, and I rushed over to see what had happened. He offered me his left elbow with a wince, explaining that he had been changing some stiff tires on his motorcycle when his grip shifted suddenly, initiating a sharp pain in his outer elbow. I was well acquainted with his tire-changing techniques, and knew that his precision engineering brain had helped him set up a system of pulleys that enabled him to apply all of his strength to pull off a recalcitrant tire without help. A "little slip" in these conditions could be quite traumatic. So far, I could see no discoloration—good. I asked him to move the elbow carefully into flexion and extension, which he was able to do without incident, and then had him move the wrist and fingers. Sure enough, actively extending the wrist produced tenderness at the elbow, as did wiggling his fingers. Static resistive testing was positive for pain and weakness of resisted wrist extension, as well as middle and ring finger extension. Then I palpated his elbow. "Arghh!" he exclaimed as he snatched the arm away from me. "That's pretty damn sore—it reminds me of the time I was playing a lot of racquetball, B.A. [before Anne] . . . back then, I couldn't even hold a coffee cup in my hand for months."

I coaxed him into letting me carefully assess his elbow once more, and as he grimaced I discovered a swollen, boggy area adjacent to the lateral epicondyle that was accompanied by a dense, hard ball of tissue that unfortunately no longer felt like it was attached. The majority of the tendon was still intact, but the freshly released fibers explained the level of his pain.

Treatment for tennis elbow is never comfortable, aside from applying modalities such as ultrasound and electrical stimulation to help reduce the localized inflammation. The bulk of hands-on therapeutic intervention consists of carefully stretching the affected muscles and tendons so they don't heal in a shortened position that will further pull against the epicondyle and re-injure the soft tissues, as well as massaging the area to improve circulation and help the healing tendon fibers to realign before initiating strengthening activities in pain free ranges of motion. Basically, touching the sore spot is like receiving a lengthy injection through a very large needle—not a recipe for warm, fuzzy husband-wife relations. "Do you want to come in to the clinic and let Jack treat your elbow?" I asked hopefully. My husband gave me The Look as I gazed back at him, discomfited. It's so difficult to hurt the ones you love! When Jack's wife had needed PT for her ankle and then later her wrist, she got onto my schedule at the clinic rather than be tortured by her own husband. Similarly, if my mother wanted to sign up for some much-needed therapy for her back, Jack would be her man. This time, it was not to be. My husband wanted my personal iron thumbs treatment, and no other. So, I commenced a series of nightly therapy sessions with the television as a distraction. "Now I know why they call you guys 'physical terrorists,'" he would grumble as I carefully but firmly applied cross-fiber friction massage to the remaining inflamed tendon fibers. It was tough to tolerate, but effective—in a few short weeks of extreme stoicism, he was back to normal, and I had been reinstated as the Best Wife in the World.

~ ★ ~

I had lost touch with Freddie after her right shoulder injury had resolved, so was surprised and worried to see her name return to my schedule two months later. Anxiously, I asked the receptionist what had happened but remained none the wiser until Freddie herself appeared, clutching her usual book, black Baggalini handbag, and bottle of water in her right hand. Her left arm dangled crookedly at her side in an attitude of stiff rejection, and she was once again without lipstick. She greeted me sheepishly, saying, "I almost felt too embarrassed to turn up here again, and nearly sneaked off to a different therapy clinic!"

"What on earth happened to you?" I exclaimed. "I mean, it's great to see you, but it would have been fine to meet at the coffee shop; there was no need to bust yourself up all over again."

Freddie said, "Well, I had a little run-in with some art supplies. I had been feeling pretty good, with my right shoulder doing so much better, and had finally decided to retire from nursing because I realized that I was getting too beat up to keep going with such an active job. You know what I mean; I would have to turn patients and reposition them in bed, stay up on my feet for long night shifts, and fiddle constantly with those overhead monitors, which was giving me a lot of issues with my neck—I am over sixty years old, you know! Anyway, I was just starting to get into the whole retirement thing and was out visiting my friend . . . we were chatting about this and that, and when I was walking past the easel she had set up for her painting, I somehow tripped over it and landed on my left arm!"

"What have you done to yourself?" I asked in apprehensive tones.

"Well, I broke my elbow in four places," she admitted awkwardly. "Now I have a plate and a bunch of screws holding it together, and the thing just won't move! So once again I can't put my hair up into a ponytail, get dressed by myself, put in earrings, or even touch my face. I need a little help!"

Poor Freddie. The saying about health professionals is so true—if something can go wrong, it will. Any doctor, nurse, or therapist who needs to have surgery is sure to encounter the maximum number of complications afterward. Freddie had not only broken her elbow spectacularly into several fragments, but the fractures had invaded the joint itself. During the initial healing process, her elbow had developed so many adhesions that it was frozen nearly solid. As per her usual response to trauma, the swelling and ecchymosis were unbelievable; it was as if she was wearing a black football around her elbow. Freddie's initial elbow passive range of motion was minus 52 degrees of extension (zero degrees, or a straight arm, being the norm) and 95 degrees of flexion (which should have been 153 degrees as compared to measurements on her "good" side). She was able to twist her wrist only 20 degrees into each direction of pronation and supination. We had our work cut out for us to bring the elbow back into a functional state.

The elbow had other ideas: when I bent it, the elbow crackled alarmingly and released waves of nauseating pain as the scar tissue wound tightly around her ulnar nerve; when I tried to straighten it, Freddie's whole shoulder would lever off the table, pinning her biceps tendon beneath the acromion in the process; and when I attempted to rotate her forearm into pronation and supination, the elbow would get stuck halfway, sending nervy zingers of pain and tingling into her wrist and fingers. It ached at rest, and screamed in agony with every attempt to mobilize the joint or stretch the soft tissues. The level of pain was intolerable, so after a hurried conference with her doctor, Freddie turned to Vicodin and then Percocet in an attempt to quiet it down enough to get it to stretch.

It was not enough. The scar tissue had set in thick and fast, giving the elbow a hard end-feel and a complete intolerance to being trifled with. At this point, Freddie's doctor decided that an elbow manipulation would be necessary. A manipulation under anesthesia is performed on a same-day surgery basis by a skilled orthopedic surgeon. Basically, the patient is put under a general anesthesia so that she is unable to fight the surgeon as he energetically pushes the joint into all of its formerly functional positions, and will feel no pain as the adhesions break apart with a resounding crack. It is essential that patients are fully relaxed and unaware, as there is a real possibility that muscles and tendons will detach from the bone as the joint is being stressed. It takes an experienced surgeon to do a good job without further damaging the joint, and only certain patients are eligible for the procedure—patients who have fractures that have not completely healed and those with osteoporosis run the risk of the bone refracturing or crumbling during the forceful intervention. Fortunately, Freddie's recent X-rays showed that her four fracture sites had healed well and were stable, so it was decided to go ahead.

I tactfully tried to prepare her for the rigors of the procedure and the expected aftermath. Because this was Freddie, we knew that her elbow would respond by swelling up monstrously afterward. Despite this outcome, it would be important for her to move her elbow as much as possible in the hours and days following the procedure in order for the elbow to stay mobile and not re-congeal. She was guardedly optimistic, and ready to move forward and start getting her life back.

The day of the procedure dawned. Freddie went off to the hospital with all my thoughts and hopes encircling her injured elbow as I anxiously awaited the outcome. When next I saw her she was pale and in pain, her elbow predictably engorged with edema and freshly black and blue. But, the elbow was finally beginning to move. "How did everything go?" I asked tentatively. Freddie smiled wanly and responded, "As well as could be expected. After the manipulation, one of the nurses spoke to me in the recovery room and said that she had felt really sorry for me in there! When my adhesions let go, there was a series of loud snapping noises that reverberated around the room."

All was well. Despite the horror of imagining poor Freddie's elbow being contorted every which way to the accompaniment of gunfire-loud noises, it was clear that a lot of progress had been made in the war against her adhesions. The end-feel of Freddie's elbow joint was now leathery instead of hard, and there was more I could do to stretch and mobilize the stiffened structures. There continued to be a thick wad of scar tissue present at her medial elbow that compressed her ulnar nerve during end range elbow flexion, but she was now able to extend her elbow to minus 35 degrees and flex it to 125 degrees. Better yet, she could now rotate her forearm almost fully, enabling her to flip her palm up and down without trouble. We still had work to do so that Freddie would be able to use the arm functionally, but she had received a flying start with the manipulation.

Freddie began to turn up to her therapy sessions with pink or red lipstick on, but still had the same pair of earrings dangling from her lobes. Progress was slow but steady. Then, late one Friday morning Freddie came in wearing a beaming smile and a bright red shirt, saying, "I can touch my face! I just can't believe it, it's been such a long time—I can actually reach my face, look!" She reached up, bending her recalcitrant elbow as much as possible to bring her fingertips to her forehead and then down her eager face to her mouth. I said, "That's fantastic! Have you tried reaching for your ear yet?" Trembling with excitement, Freddie slowly brought her left hand to her left ear with only a small amount of neck contortion. "Oh, wow," she said, "I'll be able to change my earrings now, this is fantastic!"

I said, "That's it! Tonight we'll have to celebrate with a glass of champagne."
Freddie said, "Oh no, I can't . . . we're going out with friends for dinner."

"Never mind, you can still order a glass of fizz in the restaurant," I said.
"What time are you going out? I'll raise a glass to you at the same time in a
celebratory toast."

That night at the designated time of 6:30 p.m., my husband and I faced
southwest in the direction of Freddie's restaurant and held up our glasses of
champagne in a remote toast. "To Freddie's incredible bendable elbow!" we cried
in glee. "And here's to independent ponytail setting in the near future!"

~ ★ ~

My husband had teased me for a long time about how pointed my elbows were.
He was right; my olecranon processes were rather pointy, but they served me
well, acting as sturdy buffers that prevented elbow hyperextension as I worked on
my patients. One night I beat him home after work, so started to feed our four
cats their supper while I waited for him. Because each cat was a different size, I
gave them separate bowls containing different amounts of food. Our cats were
robust eaters, and my husband and I would usually stand guard to be sure that our
largest, fastest tuxedo cat named The Pie (after the famous piebald steeplechaser in
National Velvet) wouldn't gobble his food down and then start in on Thomasina's,
Thistle's, or Koko's dinner. We had developed a feeding system so that each cat
knew which bowl was his or hers, and we had taken the extra precaution of placing a couple of large, smooth stones in The Pie's bowl around which he would
have to navigate to get all of his food. This old racehorse trick, used by some
trainers to stop the horse from gobbling his oats down at once, helped The Pie to
slow down; otherwise, a greedy Pie would end up regurgitating his supper.
Normally each cat knew its place and would eat in an orderly manner, but we
supervised them nonetheless.

That night, The Pie was ravenous and managed to scarf down his portion
while I put away the container of cat food. As I turned around, I saw him nose
Thomasina aside and start in on her bowl. "Pie, no!" I shrieked as I advanced
toward him. Unfortunately, I was wearing nothing on my feet but thick wool
socks, which skidded beneath me, allowing me to crash onto the tiled kitchen
floor directly onto my left elbow. I heard a tremendous clunk and felt instantly
nauseous as I slid across the floor. Poor Pie looked at me with a horrified expression as I ended up on my back with my feet pinning him to the wall. The rest of

the cats scattered off in divergent directions in panic, convinced that I had finally lost my mind. I lay there for a long moment, thinking desperate thoughts. Had I "done a Freddie" on myself? How would I get myself to the hospital driving my manual transmission-style car? How would I explain my foolish accident to my husband? I was sure I had fractured my elbow. As I considered my options, I moved my feet to allow the unhurt Pie to escape and then I heard my husband pull into the driveway. I couldn't let him see me like this! Groaning, I hauled myself to my feet and began to assess the situation. The elbow looked normal. Gingerly, I tried to move it a little, and then a little more. It was OK! Unbelievable. I hurriedly thanked my strapping, well-built ancestors and moved forward to greet my husband with outstretched arms.

Unfortunately, my ancestors still had something to answer for. Despite the sturdiness of my elbows, the muscles surrounding them had an alarming tendency to tighten and thicken in response to the hard manual labor that was involved in the delivery of hands-on physical therapy treatment. Over time I had noticed a low-grade tingling sensation in my left wrist and fingers that I suspected was carpal tunnel syndrome, but as it remained at a dull roar, I simply tuned it out and kept going with life. Then, I signed up for a continuing education course on the neural tension of peripheral nerves, the nerves that connect the brain and spinal cord, or central nervous system (CNS), to the rest of the body. The peripheral nerves are composed of outgoing motor fibers, which carry electrical impulses from the CNS to the muscles to ask them to perform a contraction, and of incoming sensory nerves, which deliver messages about pain and pressure occurring at the limbs to the CNS. Peripheral nerves are notoriously fussy and delicate to treat as nerve tissue is nonstretchy and unforgiving to pressure. Neural tissue is like a piece of dental floss—it slides easily, but when stretched, it does not regain its shape; with enough stretching force, it will break.

When a nerve is either stretched or compressed, it lets you know about it in a hurry, grumpily becoming oversensitized and producing a lot of tingling and numbness anywhere along the neural pathway. Although the nerves will frequently exhibit a deep, aching pain sensation directly over the site of compression, they also send burning, stabbing, or sharp pains anywhere along their length. This tendency is a constant source of aggravation to dedicated doctors and therapists, who can only guess at the original site of nerve injury based on the onset of symptoms, the aggravating and relieving factors, and the pattern of pain. The ultimate tests to determine the source of a peripheral nerve injury are to perform a nerve conduction velocity (NCV) test with electromyography (EMG).

Nerve conduction studies are designed to measure the function of the motor and sensory peripheral nerves, giving information about potential sites and degrees of compression or stretch. Nerve compression may be localized, such as occurs with an entrapment syndrome like carpal tunnel syndrome of the wrist, or may be widespread, as with a diabetic neuropathy in which the feet and even the entire lower legs may be affected. With a nerve overstretch or compression injury, the sensory parts of the nerves are usually affected first, causing tingling and numbness of the affected extremity. If the area remains compressed, the nerve becomes sticky and will no longer slide normally among the surrounding tissues, the motor fibers also become injured, and weakness results in the muscles supplied by that nerve.

Of course, the curative treatment is to help decompress the affected nerves and to assist the swollen and inflamed neural tissue to glide normally once more. The continuing education course I signed up for was to review techniques of peripheral nervous system mobilization that would assist in this delicate process of recovery. I was excited to attend the course and had high hopes that I would be able to learn a new technique to help me cure my tingling hand.

The first rule of treating nervous tissues is to Exercise Extreme Caution. Nerves are fragile, easily injured tissues, and once injured they have a disturbing tendency to heal with agonizing slowness or not at all. Despite having this knowledge, enthusiastic therapists easily can cause pain to their patients or even themselves. As usual, I threw myself into the course material with great gusto, keen to review the strategies and even keener to see if I could sort out my wonky hand. All was well until we reached the final exercises in which we were to practice self-mobilization techniques on ourselves. We all lay down as instructed in various relaxed attitudes on our towels on the floor and proceeded to follow the instructor's directions. We gradually increased the tension on our own upper extremity neural tissues by first depressing our shoulder blades, then bringing our affected bent arm away from our sides, then progressively straightening the elbow and extending the wrist and fingers. This action was designed to take up the slack in our neural tissues running from the cervical nerve roots to our fingertips, and was to be repeated in a pumping action in order to slide the nerves throughout the arm. Unfortunately, I had extreme neural tension in my left arm that began with step one, depressing the shoulder blade. Undeterred, the instructor advised me to continue with the entire exercise despite my deeply painful symptoms, and my nerves became well and truly stretched. Now I had burning pain, tingling, and numbness in my left ring and little finger in addition to my wrist, and had learned an expensive cautionary tale—we never know what lies beneath a "normal looking" arm.

Months and then years went by, and my symptoms continued unabated. I became convinced that I had injured my ulnar nerve at its origins somewhere in my neck, because I also began experiencing neck pain and increased symptoms when looking down at my patients around that time. Finally I sought help from a physiatrist, and underwent an NCV test with EMG. The NCV test is performed using surface electrodes that deliver and then measure a mild electrical impulse as it travels between the two points. The speed of nerve conduction is measured and compared to the unaffected side and to standardized normative values. The location of nerve compression or injury can be pinpointed according to where the slowed nerve conduction or diminished response occurs, as measured over different segments of the nerve. To my surprise, the test localized a segment of compression at my left elbow, and not my neck after all. There was also an area of compression at the wrist (moderate carpal tunnel syndrome), but I had already become used to that and it was not progressing.

Then, Dr. G moved on to perform the EMG. This is a slightly painful procedure, since it involves the insertion of a sterile needle into the muscles of the arm. The muscle activity is measured at rest and then upon my active muscular contraction (this was the painful part!) to compare the signals. Dr. G had recently been in a bicycling accident and had given himself a spectacular road rash on his right leg, hip, and buttock, so was perched uneasily on the rolling stool beside me as he reached for my elbow with the needle. My first clue came when Dr. G couldn't get the needle into my arm just below the elbow. After a fair amount of sweating and cursing, he commented, "No wonder you've got ulnar nerve entrapment—your muscles and fascia are thicker than a day laborer's!" Finally, he inserted the needle with a nasty pop as it pierced my toughened fascia. "That's it!" he exclaimed. "Cubital tunnel syndrome. This is all abnormal . . . does it ache at night? Do you drop things? Is the tingling constant?" (Yes, yes, and yes).

I was happy to identify the problem, but less than thrilled with the diagnosis. Apparently my stint at the continuing education course had accelerated the friction of the ulnar nerve against my already tight forearm muscles, exacerbating a problem that had been building up for years. Over time, with the delivery of thousands of hands-on treatments, my ulnar nerve had less and less room to glide and ended up getting squeezed in the elbow groove as surely as if my nerve was a garden hose that someone was standing on while I was trying to water my plants. It was likely that I had built up fibrous scar tissue in the area that could be helped by surgery, but I knew from my patient care experiences that surgical decompression of the ulnar nerve could be extremely simple but also fraught with peril, the neural tissues being so delicate. My only other options included anti-inflammatory modalities, myofascial release techniques, careful nerve gliding, and relentless continual repositioning of the elbow to avoid further compression.

After months of conservative self-imposed physical therapy, the motor component of my ulnar nerve improved and my strength returned so that I stopped dropping things, such as my keys, at odd moments; however, my sensory symptoms diminished but did not abate. I continued to feel constant tingling twenty-four hours a day, seven days a week, that would escalate to a deep, toothache-like pain whenever my elbow was bent too long or if I had to use my left arm with any significant force upon my patients. However, I knew that once an organism has been cut into surgically, there are no guarantees for success, especially with such a long-standing injury. Once scar tissue has formed, even the best surgeon can try to remove it but has no control over the individual body's responses to re-form the scar tissue; in fact, things may end up worse than before. I have resigned myself to lifelong left elbow and hand tingling, but recognize that its presence makes me even more sensitive to my patients' plight. Sadly, not everything once damaged can be fixed. I learned a valuable lesson: to listen to my body when it whispers to me, so I don't have to hear the eventual screams.

With a Twist of the Wrist

The difference between a helping hand and an outstretched palm is a twist of the wrist.

—*Laurence Leamer, author and Kennedy family biographer (1941–)*

When we look down at our wrists, we see a simple structure where the telltale skin creases denote a region of supple movement. However, the wrist is no plain hinge joint but is made up of many articulations between eight carpal bones, the ends of the radius and ulna that originate at the elbow, and the five metacarpal bones of the fingers. It is this snug jigsaw puzzle of carpal bones that gives the wrist its extreme maneuverability and allows us to transform the gross movements of the upper body into the delicate, finely coordinated manipulations of the hand and fingers.

At first blush, the wrist just seems like a bag of old bones thrown as haphazardly together as if they had tumbled randomly out of some voodoo doctor's magic bag. The carpal bones are irregularly shaped and awkward, and I found it difficult to remember the name and orientation of each bone until I learned an age-old mnemonic in PT school. I discovered that if I looked at the palm side of my left wrist, I could divide the mysterious chunks of bone roughly into two rows and "read" them from left to right. Beginning with the row closest to my heart, I could recite, "Some lovers try positions that they can't handle." This neatly correlated to the scaphoid, lunate, triquetrum, pisiform, trapezium, trapezoid, capitate, and hamate. Easy!

The carpal bones move in a coordinated, complex series of jostling slips and slides to allow global wrist joint movement. Despite being held into place by a series of strong ligaments, the carpals are able to slightly shift against each other as the overlying tendons pull on the hand and forearm (only the flexor carpi ulnaris tendon actually inserts directly into the pisiform; the rest simply glide past within the carpal tunnel). The vast majority of wrist movement is made possible by movements of the proximal carpal bones against the radius. Amazingly, there is no direct articulation between the ulna and the carpal bones; rather, the stubby end of the ulna is buffered away from the proximal carpal row by a large triangle of cartilage (triangular fibrocartilage complex).

The majority of accidents that end in wrist fractures or dislocations involve a fall onto the outstretched hand, either during sports activities or when one experiences an accidental loss of balance. Although fractures are nothing to trifle with and are amazingly inconvenient during the recovery phase, they are often easier to heal than soft tissue injuries are. In the wrist, the most well-known, highly publicized soft tissue injury that plagues thousands of patients each year is carpal tunnel syndrome. The infamous carpal tunnel is merely a space within the wrist that lies between the carpal bones and a restraining band made of fibrous connective tissue that keeps the tendons from popping away from the wrist during flexion. Within the tunnel lie nine flexor tendons, several blood vessels, and the median nerve. When the tendons traveling within the carpal tunnel are repeatedly frictioned back and forth against the carpal bones and the fibrous restraining band like ropes slipping through the hands of a tug-of-war team, they become inflamed and swell. When they swell, they fill the space of the carpal tunnel and crowd out their neighbors (the median nerve and blood vessels), resulting in pain and tingling. Despite the controversy that blames most cases of carpal tunnel syndrome on poor ergonomics at the workstation, carpal tunnel syndrome is more likely to result from poor positioning, repetitive motions, certain primary diseases, pregnancy, or direct wrist trauma.

As they watch me work on them, patients repeatedly ask me if I have trouble with my own wrists. Physical therapists are no strangers to injury because of the manual nature of our work, but we can become role models for some of our struggling wrist patients by sensible example. The secret to maintaining happy wrists is to use them sparingly and in a variety of positions. Whenever I need to massage or mobilize one of my patients in ways that force my wrists into end range extension, I make sure that I change my wrist and hand positions frequently. This allows the circulation to return to compressed tendons, muscles, and nerves, allowing the soft tissues to recover and reducing the chance of injury.

~ ★ ~

The wrist is a living road map to human evolution that shows us the progress of changing DNA. An interesting place to see this is in the palmar surface of the wrist. When you hold the wrist in a slightly flexed position and then touch the thumb to the little finger, you can see the tendon of palmaris longus pop out against the surface skin. This muscle is estimated to be absent in up to 25 percent of the population, and it is thought that given more time, the muscle will eventually be extinguished from the human race. This assumption is based on the overwhelming presence of palmaris longus in lower apes, such as the orangutan, versus a much lower incidence of the muscle in higher apes, such as chimpanzees. (I have a palmaris longus tendon in my right wrist, but not in my left—am I only partially evolved?)

Because of its small size, noticeable length, and ancillary role as an ineffective wrist flexor, the palmaris longus is a relatively nonessential body part that can be harvested for use as a tendon graft to restore ruptured tendons in the hand. Regardless, humans did not evolve to sit still for long. We just weren't designed to hunch over hot computers in positions of near immobility for hours on end with our wrists cocked at odd angles, nor were we supposed to stand and repeatedly perform the same motions over and over, steadily building up friction on our swelling tendons. The human body likes movement and variety, and thrives on frequent position changes, handholds, and postures.

~ ★ ~

I chose my first PT job carefully after graduating from the master's program and passing the national board examination. My goal was to keep learning in an environment of seasoned therapists, so that if I lacked confidence in a certain diagnosis, disease, or condition, I would have a good support system. This was not only to help me transition from the student life to the professional life, but also to protect my patients from harm. I decided to work in a busy outpatient clinic near a large hospital that offered a reasonable amount of money for formal continuing education course work each year, and where there were ten other physical and occupational therapists busily treating patients. It was a paradise of mentors.

The only drawback to the clinic was that the line between physical and occupational therapy was razor sharp—the PTs were not allowed to treat wrist, hand, or finger patients because there was a certified hand therapist (who happened to be an occupational therapist, or OT) onboard. After some settling-in time, I asked to be allowed to observe and occasionally treat a hand patient in order to further expand my confidence and skills. Fortunately, this wish was granted, so if I had an empty patient slot during the day I could walk over to the west side of the building to watch the OTs in action.

The second-in-command OT, Kristen, was a willowy blonde with long hair, long legs, startlingly blue eyes, and a practical nature. She had skilled hands and a dry wit that facilitated easy, informal relationships with her patients, a trait I envied in my raw, inexperienced state. I was still a little cautious and anxious about my approach and hand placement when working with my own patients, and I was in awe of her; besides, Kristen had six whole years of patient care under her belt. I could hardly wait to gain that degree of experience and the confidence it brings.

Kristen always welcomed me with a casual nod of her head from her position hunched over a patient's hand. The cases were interesting, consisting of a mixture of postsurgical tendon transfers, finger reattachments following accidental amputation, and of course our bread-and-butter friend, carpal tunnel syndrome. One sunny afternoon I happened upon the hand clinic just as Kristen was greeting a new patient, Harry, for the first time. As I introduced myself and got comfortably seated on a nearby stool, Harry explained that he worked more than fourteen hours a day on the computer in a Silicon Valley start-up firm and that over time he had developed carpal tunnel syndrome in his right hand. It had become so bad that he had agreed to have the local hand surgery expert perform a carpal tunnel release, in which the fibrous connective tissue restraining band is resected to decompress the median nerve beneath. Harry was now in the postoperative phase, and had been sent to the therapy clinic to help him decrease his wrist swelling and to regain his range of motion and strength.

As I looked on, Kristen began to assess the degree of stiffness and swelling in Harry's right wrist. At the same time, I could see Harry examining Kristen with equal alacrity. Then, he brought up the topic of movies, specifically James Bond films, and waxed poetic about some of the starring Bond girls he had especially liked over the years. Sure enough, his taste leaned toward the blondes, particularly Honor Blackman. While Kristen bent low over Harry's wrist, carefully measuring the circumferential swelling around his recovering wrist, Harry described the faux hay fight between Ms. Blackman and Sean Connery in the movie *Goldfinger* with great relish. As I smiled to myself, enjoying Harry's thinly disguised flirting with Kristen (who steadfastly ignored his overtures and focused professionally on his wrist), Harry burst out, "Kristen, can I call you 'Pussy Galore'?" Kristen calmly shot back, "No, you can't . . . now, does this hurt?" as she gently squeezed his incision. Harry squirmed a little and stopped flirting, behaving himself like a gentleman from that moment on. Kristen could have excelled as a poker player, and I learned a lot from her about maintaining a deadpan expression of professional interest, giving no visible reaction during the times when patients wanted to wind me up.

~ ★ ~

Sarah staggered into the clinic grimly clutching her husband's arm, her gaze fixed numbly on the floor and her narrow face pale and clammy. Her tortured expression was drawn with pain, and she held her left wrist stiffly as it peeked out from the protective burrow of her navy blue arm sling. Sarah whispered for a cup of water before collapsing into a nearby chair, shaking with apprehension. Her husband explained that they had just come back from a visit to the anesthesiologist, who had tried a sympathetic nerve block in Sarah's neck in an effort to "turn off" her reflex sympathetic dystrophy (RSD). Also known as complex regional pain syndrome, RSD is a chronic condition that is thought to come from sympathetic nervous system dysfunction. This intensely painful problem usually happens to an arm or leg after a major injury has occurred; somehow, central and/or peripheral pain receptors become overly sensitized to certain nerve chemicals and flood the affected area with severe pain, joint stiffness, muscle spasms, and skin changes. Typical symptoms include an excruciating, burning pain that is out of proportion to the original injury; reddened or purplish skin color; shiny, extremely sensitive skin; swelling; changes in local skin temperature and sweatiness; and changes in the nail and hair growth patterns of the extremity. Any increase in emotional stress will exacerbate the already unbearable symptoms. Basically, RSD is a living hell for the sufferer, an inexplicable pain that is present without reason or mercy.

Sarah had originally broken her wrist in a fall onto her outstretched arm when she had lost her balance over a bit of uneven sidewalk on the way to church. Her injury was a classic Colles' fracture, in which the end of the distal radius had been broken. Because the radius normally rotates around the ulna to provide supination and pronation, Sarah's wrist had to be pinned into place to avoid displacement of the bone fragments while they healed. A fixated fracture is a stable fracture, but until healing was complete and the pins removed, Sarah was unable to twist her wrist at all. Furthermore, she admitted to having an extremely poor pain tolerance and had not even tried to move her hand or fingers during the initial recovery phase. By the time I saw her, the wrist was like a shiny, exquisitely painful piece of ice.

Her wrist could not be touched at all, even with the lightest pressure. Sarah had been sleeping with her left arm on top of the comforter for fear of the bedclothes inadvertently touching her skin at night. She could not bear a gentle breeze to cross the delicate hairs on her forearm, and had resolutely refused to even look at the wrist for weeks. In desperation, her surgeon had sent her to receive PT at another clinic but since Sarah couldn't tolerate even the briefest contact on her wrist, the experiment was abandoned. Instead, the surgeon ordered a series of sympathetic nerve injections via the neck to block the flow generated by the sympathetic nerves into the upper extremity. Immediately following the block, she was to come over for another attempt at PT, this time with me.

I escorted Sarah and her husband back to the treatment room, made her comfortable in the chair, and placed a small paper cup of water so that it was readily available to her right hand. Then I started looking at her left wrist. It was red, shiny, and stiffly held in a neutral position, halfway between pronation and supination. When I asked her to try moving the wrist and fingers, she had no luck. It was as if the whole arm belonged to a department store mannequin. I carefully tried contacting her forearm proximal to her wrist with a butterfly touch, using hand lotion to lubricate her skin and reduce the friction between us. Sarah handled it with tightly closed eyes and a grimace as I gently worked my way down toward her wrist. Her husband said, "Wow, that's a lot better!" as I lightly passed over her wrist and hand. I chatted about nothing in particular and attempted to distract her with naughty pet stories (they had cats at home, too), when Sarah finally spoke. "I can't believe you're touching my wrist!" she whispered faintly. "This is great—there's hope after all. I've been feeling so upset by everything, and seem to cry constantly about my wrist, my life, and the state of the world . . . nothing's been the same for me since 9/11."

"Oh, I'm so sorry," I said as I slightly shook my head, experiencing one of my lightheaded moments. "Did you lose someone in the World Trade Center or on Flight 93 or at the Pentagon?"

"No . . . it's just the worry that something else will happen. What will I do if a plane flies into the Transamerica Pyramid in San Francisco? How can I protect myself and my family? How can . . ."

I caught her upper body in my arms as she fainted, slumping sideways in her chair. Sarah came to almost immediately, apologizing for her lapse. I comforted her, explaining that despite the nerve block her body remained on high alert and was poised for flight even if she was unable to physically escape. The pain in her arm, combined with a feeling of being out of control both physically and mentally, was simply too much for her system to handle. Furthermore, her entire lower arm from the elbow to the fingertips needed to be desensitized before I could continue with the odious task of mobilizing her wrist joint and restoring normal range of motion. So, I prescribed a home exercise program for her, consisting of a series of progressive stimuli to her forearm, wrist, and hand that would gradually remove the alarming sympathetic nervous system response and desensitize the skin. I asked Sarah to begin by touching her wrist gently with an extremely light material such as a silk scarf, progressively repeating the frequency and duration of the contact. Then, when this was more tolerable she was to use rougher and more textured materials such as cotton, linen, wool, and even Velcro against all the surfaces of her skin. From this point, she could start to use gentle and then firm pressure, warm then cool temperatures, and light vibration; eventually she could try pressing through her hand and wrist in positions of gentle weight bearing.

Sarah made tremendous progress in a very short period of time and I was soon able to touch and then to delicately mobilize and stretch her fingers, elbow, and hand, working my way gradually inward toward the wrist. Her home program changed to emphasize asking her left hand and wrist to participate in functional tasks; for example, when drinking a cup of water, Sarah was no longer to ignore her left hand and wrist but instead to engage it in pantomiming and then following the right hand's actions. When she reached out with her right hand to adjust her glasses, she was to bring both hands to her face, using the left side in conjunction with the right as naturally as possible. Throughout her normal activities of daily living, Sarah was to focus on standing and sitting up with good posture to reduce the amount of compensatory protective slumping that can lead to muscle guarding of the affected extremity. Once she had a definite plan, Sarah brightened up considerably. But she still had a long way to go in her recovery and regretted not yet being able to wear her wedding band. "The priest placed my wedding ring on my finger, and I vowed never to take it off," she said.

"Sadly, when I fractured my wrist my entire hand and fingers swelled up so badly that the nurses in emergency made me remove it, threatening me that if I didn't that they would cut it off! Now I still wear it, but have to keep it here instead," she said as she reached into her neckline with her right hand to lift out the plain wedding band that lay threaded onto a simple gold chain.

Since her wrist movement had been restricted for a long period of time following surgery and Sarah had completely dissociated herself from her left hand and wrist, I knew that the position sensors (proprioceptors) of the wrist would be damaged. Joking that it would now be therapeutic for Sarah to help her husband wash his car, I encouraged her to perform tasks where she would need to press some of her weight through her hand and wrist, giving the joints much-needed proprioceptive stimulation.

"My car's never been cleaner!" Sarah's husband laughed the next time they came into the clinic. "But seriously, I've noticed that during the night Sarah keeps her left arm tucked in under the covers now, and can see that she's trying real hard to use the wrist more . . . she's a real trooper."

"I'm so glad to hear that you're able to use the wrist more; but how is the pain?" I asked Sarah.

She said, "Well, it's actually getting a little more comfortable; it seems like the more I use it (within reason!), the better it gets. As you can see, it's still swollen, but it's definitely less red, and the burning feeling isn't nearly as intense. My biggest problem is that I have no ability to grip anything with my left hand; pulling on my underwear is a real chore! The other problem is that my wrist is my whole life. I'm constantly thinking about it, working on it, and feeling it. I'm getting forgetful about anything else."

"Don't feel bad," I said. "Brain overload can do that to a person, and it's happened to me, too. One day I was especially busy, racing from pillar to post between my patients, doctor phone calls, insurance company requests, progress notes, and office management issues. I finally sprinted out of here at the eleventh hour to go for my routine dental cleaning (he won't see me if I'm late), and made it with two minutes to spare. Recognizing a golden opportunity to use the bathroom, I popped in to the restroom and quickly availed myself of the facilities, only to find out that I'd made it all the way through the day with my underwear turned inside out! How's that for forgetfulness?!"

And so it went. As the sensitivity and swelling decreased, I was able to help Sarah regain her range of motion by progressively mobilizing her wrist joints and stretching out the contracted tendons. Finally, a special day arrived. Smiling broadly, Sarah greeted me with a triumphant expression, dangling her left hand in front of my face. "Look, look—do you notice anything different?" she asked. There it was, back in its rightful position at last—Sarah's wedding ring glowed in triumph on her fourth finger.

~ ★ ~

Not all of the spooky, intuitive moments that involve healing have happened with patient care. One very wet late spring day found me taking my exuberant gray horse, Atlas, to a local trainer to help me give him more experience in crowded environments. Until that time, Atlas's reaction to new surroundings and strange horses was to attempt to mimic the flying leaps of the world-renowned Spanish riding school Lipizzaner stallions. Atlas's antics not only made it difficult for the rider to sit, but also they could be dangerous, as on occasion he would become so keyed up that he would end up falling down on his side in the mud. So, I would ride him a mile down the road to the local riding school each weekend, where we worked on desensitization of his emotional outbursts. Atlas steadily improved but was still prone to flinging out a few errant bucks and leaps, showing off, if he got too close to another horse. However, I was well pleased with his progress. But, after that very rainy spring day in which he actually managed to keep all of his feet on the ground, Atlas turned up lame. It was a total mystery. He seemed comfortable enough standing and walking around, but when asked to move out into a trot or canter, he was clearly unsound in his left front leg.

My therapist's eye is fairly keen when it comes to assessing movement disorders in people and animals, but this time I simply could not localize the problem. I poked and prodded Atlas all over, but was unable to find any swelling, tender spot, or cut. Nothing appeared to be wrong, but at any pace faster than a slow walk Atlas was head-bobbing lame. When a day or so of watchful waiting showed no improvement, I trudged off to call my veterinarian. We tried every test in the book—palpation, nerve block injections, and flexion tests (in which the horse's limbs are systematically flexed for one minute to stress the ligaments and then the horse is asked to trot off—a positive test is one that temporarily worsens the lameness), but to no avail. Nothing triggered a response, and Atlas limped on just the same. My veterinarian was stumped. I was stumped. Days and weeks passed without change. The problem was definitely somewhere in Atlas's left front leg, but it was impossible to know if the pain was originating in his shoulder, elbow, knee (the horse's "wrist," which is the location of the carpal bones), ankle, or foot.

Despite his lameness I continued to visit Atlas each day to feed him, pet him, comfort him, and test his soundness, but nothing changed. Finally, a good friend said over coffee, "Why don't you contact my pet psychic? I'll bet she could tell you where the problem is!" This sort of comment does me little good, since as a Western-trained health professional I remain highly skeptical of anything unproven or that I cannot see concretely for myself, let alone attempt to visualize in the abstract. At this time Atlas was just a young horse, and although I was frantic to help him feel better, I had little idea how. Instead, I arranged to take Atlas to the famous UC Davis veterinary medicine teaching hospital, where they could perform a nuclear scan on him to help finally localize the problem area, allowing treatment to begin. Nuclear scintigraphy is a form of bone scanning that is able to highlight areas of inflamed or damaged tissues via injecting radioactive markers into the bloodstream. The horse is then scanned for "hot spots" where the radioactive compound is being taken up the fastest by injured cells with rapid turnover rates. Because any tissue with a blood supply (such as muscle, tendon, ligament, or bone) will take up the radioactive compound, an occult area of injury can be identified. At this point, it was my only chance to find out where Atlas was hurting, since he couldn't tell me himself.

But, I couldn't get an appointment for the nuclear scan until the following week. With a mounting sense of desperation and a feeling of helplessness (what if Atlas was irrevocably damaging himself in the interim?) I called my friend to get the pet psychic's phone number. I had nothing to lose. The consultation was thirty dollars for fifteen minutes, during which time you were to describe your pet's appearance and where the pet lived so that the psychic could "talk" to your pet while she looked at a map to help channel her energy. If there was enough lead-in time, you could also send a photograph to help the psychic center her mind on the pet. Since I noticed that the psychic also lived in California, I quickly sent a photo of Atlas off and made an appointment for the following day. I told no one, not even my husband, for fear of sounding like a total nutcase.

The next day I hunched over my cell phone and called the psychic while sitting on Atlas's feed container in his paddock. I told her Atlas's name, age, and breed, but gave her no particular reason for my consultation. In my attempt to "test" her, the photo I had sent showed Atlas standing alone in front of his stable with no other horses in sight. The first thing the psychic said was, "Atlas wants to know what happened to his friend." I was speechless, my mind racing. I said,

"What does he mean?" She responded, "His friend, the chestnut gelding with the white face and white socks who used to live next to him . . . he wants to know what happened to the other horse."

The small hairs stood up on the nape of my neck and chills trickled down my spine as I looked at Atlas, munching his hay without apparent concern. His next-door neighbor, Monty, was a chestnut American Quarter Horse with a white face and legs who had recently been sold due to chronic lameness. Monty had left the stables just the month before when his uncaring owner had suddenly decided to get rid of him. There was no way the psychic could have known what Atlas's old neighbor looked like. Things were getting pretty weird. I told her what had happened to Monty and waited for more. The psychic went on, "Oh, okay—Atlas just wanted to know. Now, he's telling me that he doesn't like his salt block. You have one of those pinkish ones, the ones with the trace minerals, right? He says he just wants one that's pure salt, one of the plain white ones."

Again I started in surprise as Atlas chewed on unconcernedly beside me. He did have the trace mineral salt block, and yes, it was pink. I assured the psychic that I would get him a new one. Then she said, "He keeps telling me that his left front leg is bothering him. Have you noticed any lameness? Because he says that his left leg is hurting."

I said, "Yes, I've been worried about his leg; in fact, that's really why I called. Where exactly does he say it hurts?"

"It's behind his left knee. It looks like he sprained some ligaments back there . . . he keeps taking me to the back of his left knee. He says it's not real serious and he hasn't wanted to worry you, but it's bothering him. Aside from that, he says he's pretty happy, and he likes the bay horse a lot; the bay is his best friend."

The bay horse was the only other horse at the small family-owned stables where I kept Atlas. The bay was my other horse, Riley, and he and Atlas were good friends who always played together, usually to the exclusion of the recently departed Monty. It was all very strange. After the consultation was over, I palpated the back of Atlas's left knee with renewed vigor. Nothing. Could she be right? I had no clue. Plus, how was I to tell my vet that a psychic instructed me that Atlas had sprained the suspensory ligaments behind his carpals? I decided to keep my nuclear scan appointment.

Having cleared my patient schedule for the afternoon of the scan, I set out to make the ninety-mile journey to Davis with Atlas riding behind me in our horse trailer. Unfortunately, the temperatures were soaring above 100 degrees, and neither one of us was happy. I had to keep the air conditioner turned off in the truck to preserve engine power to pull the weight of Atlas and the trailer without overheating, and Atlas himself had only the breeze of the road to cool him as he rode along. After an unpleasant journey, part of which was accomplished in the stirrings of rush hour traffic and with a few miles spent in tandem with a smelly rendering truck (poor Atlas!) we arrived at the veterinary hospital. They would perform the scan right away, but would have to keep Atlas overnight in order to monitor him until all of the radioactivity had left his system. I settled down to wait.

When the results came in, I was happy to have a definitive diagnosis, but I didn't know what to think. The scan showed that Atlas had pulled a suspensory ligament in the back of his left knee. It was a classic "wrist sprain," with a treatment plan of nonsteroidal anti-inflammatories, massage to stimulate the circulation, rest, and careful strengthening before his return to work, just like in the PT clinic. In time, Atlas recovered without incident, but I continue to wonder. My mind has been wrenched open as to the possibilities of all the things that can't be seen with our eyes or proven with science.

Reaching Out to the Light

Dare to reach out your hand into the darkness, to pull another hand into the light.

—*Norman B. Rice, first African American mayor of Seattle, Washington (1943–)*

The role of the physical therapist is to fix things—broken bodies, uneasy minds, and interrupted lives. As we learn our craft, therapists soon figure out that it takes a firm yet light touch combined with lots of encouragement to help people regain their former levels of function. Yet, it is not always possible to return to exactly what went before.

The hand is one of the most delicate and sensitive structures to work with, and is the repository of the patient's past and present history. Knuckles may be swollen with hard work or rheumatoid arthritis. Fingers can be bent, deformed, or twisted from previous injury. The skin on the back of the hand might look spotted with age, wrinkled from dehydration, or puffy from underlying swelling. Hands are extremely expressive, and often communicate invaluable information unbeknownst to their owners. Sometimes, the hands are the last parts of us to stop working, even when all is lost.

~ ★ ~

My father's hands sported sparse fingernails from his habitual nail biting, early age spots from too much sunbathing, and a plain, white gold wedding band that was slowly disappearing into his flesh. He had fought his lymphoma with gusto for many years and had earned a five-year respite during which he was able to attend my PT school graduation, walk me down the aisle, and see his last grandchild enter the world. He packed as much living as possible into the waning moments of his life, finally succumbing to liver failure as the chemotherapy chose to kill him, beating his cancer to the finish line.

Our immediate family stayed with my father in the hospital as he railed against his fate, slipping in and out of consciousness as his liver slowly gave in to toxicity. At first we were able to talk and reminisce, but he gradually began to fade toward a distant, shimmering road that only he could see. Sadly, with all my medical knowledge, there was nothing I could do other than try to help my family recognize what was to come. My mother, brother, and I kept vigil as my father struggled to stay with us. I had looked up the signs of end stage liver failure and knew that part of the process would involve involuntary grimaces, violent seizures, and flapping movements of the hands.

As his final night faded into the gray dawn, I tried to keep hold of my father's hand, knowing that such a volatile, vibrant, selfish, gregarious, frustrating, friendly, outrageous man wouldn't want to be alone in his hour of need. As morning broke, all four of us were still breathing, but the hand flapping became more intense as the seizures worsened, my father now deep in his coma. In desperation we each in turn spoke our final farewells, hoping that he could still hear us.

Just before we began a prayer for him, my father's two doctors came in to check on his status and graciously fell into a circle around his hospital bed as we held hands together around my father's struggling form. When the final "Amen" sounded, I felt a shaft of fearful certainty pierce my heart as my father began his worst seizure yet, his hands moving wildly; then, the flapping hand movements mercifully stopped as he slipped away to freedom.

~ ★ ~

I had been working with Roger for several weeks to mobilize his stiff left shoulder and strengthen his rotator cuff muscles. He had been making excellent progress, but then mysteriously disappeared from my schedule for two weeks. No one seemed to know what had happened, and although we had left him messages on his home answering machine, he had not returned our calls. When Roger finally returned to the clinic, he was wearing a thick white gauze bandage on his left hand and index finger.

"Whatever happened to you?" I asked with concern. "We were worried—didn't you get our messages?"

"Yeah, well you know since I haven't been able to work the machines at my job because of my shoulder healing, I've been doing more supervisory stuff. I was helping one of my guys figure out one of the jammed pieces of equipment a couple of weeks ago, when my finger got caught in it! Man, it was ugly . . . but good thing it wasn't my middle finger! They made me go and see the work doctor, who had me stay away from therapy until the finger started to heal, since it's on the same arm as my hurt shoulder," he said.

"Do you feel up to me working on your shoulder today? I promise to be careful and not jostle your finger!" I said.

"Sure! I've missed all the torture," he replied.

After checking out Roger's shoulder range of motion and noting that he still had an arc of impingement from 90 degrees to 120 degrees of shoulder abduction when moving his arm away from his body, I set to work on loosening the shoulder up. As I performed some inferior glides on his glenohumeral joint, I flashed on an image of our black cat, Thomasina, turning up her nose at a bowl of cereal milk. My husband and I always joke that Thomasina is so sensitive that she should be hired as a royal taste tester, since she was always the first to notice if the milk was beginning to spoil. I thought, that's odd . . . why would I think of my cat during a treatment? I mentally shook myself, and turned my full attention back to Roger's shoulder.

But then, the image returned and I started to imagine that I could smell mold. "Roger, do you smell anything funny in here?" I asked.

"No, I swear I showered and put deodorant on before I came over!" he joked.

Hmm. Something wasn't quite right. I asked, "When was the last time you saw your 'finger doctor'?"

"It's been about a week," he replied. "Everything was looking pretty good, so he just told me to keep it clean and dry and to go back to see him at the end of next week."

I reached down and gently lifted his bandaged hand. Now I could smell the moldy aroma more strongly. "Roger, do you mind if we take a peek at this? You might need to change the dressing or something—it seems a little ripe," I said.

"Peek away," he said. "I haven't seen it for awhile, so let's check it out."

I carefully removed his intricate gauze bandage, the smell becoming more intense with each unfolded layer. Horrified, I could see that his finger was not healing normally but was becoming blackened and necrotic, the rotting tissues clearly being the source of the putrid smell. Not wanting to alarm him, I said, "Roger, I think that you need a new bandage right away. This one is getting pretty stinky . . . can you stop by your finger doctor's office after therapy today? I think he should see it and make sure it's healing OK—it doesn't look quite right to me."

Roger agreed, so we rewrapped the finger and I quickly finished our session. I called his doctor and waited on tenterhooks for our next visit, worrying about Roger's finger, until I was finally rewarded by seeing his name on my schedule again the following week.

Roger had already been shown into a treatment room, so at his appointment time I knocked and entered. No Roger. Then, out of the corner of my eye I saw him ease toward me from behind the door and was surprised to feel a soft kiss planted on my cheek. "Thank you for saving my finger," he said as he held a hand-blown glass flower out to me. "You were right. After I left here, I went to see my doctor, who rushed me in for surgery on my finger. He said I had gangrene, and even though he cleaned it up and I lost some flesh for good, he was able to save the finger. Look . . ."

Roger carefully unwrapped his left index finger, freeing it from its bulky bandage. There, even though part of the side and tip of his finger was gone, I could see new healthy tissue gleaming beneath the antibacterial ointment. Surreptitiously, I sniffed the surrounding air—nothing. All was well again, with no more finicky cat images coming to mind.

~ ★ ~

A person's hands can tell you a lot about them. My hands are noticeably care-worn and bear the scars of myriad outdoor activities and patient care–related moments. The nails are clipped short and tidy on a weekly basis, with only a scant amount of white fingernail tip showing—this practice keeps me from accidentally scratching my patients as I work on them, reduces the bacterial burden that could potentially infect my patients' wounds, and also protects me from inadvertently gathering my patients' skin cells beneath my fingernails, a thought that makes me shudder. The left index finger sports a crooked scar and twisted interphalangeal joint where the impact of a speeding bicyclist cleaved my knuckle during my undergraduate days at UC Davis, and the little finger shows an old, thin slash where my brother accidentally nearly pruned the last joint off in our garden during childhood. The left ring finger is pale and narrowed at the base from the comforting pressure of wearing my wedding ring for well over a decade. There is a matching red discoloration on the right ring finger from the time I deeply scraped off all the skin when I accidentally trapped it between a treatment table and the clinic wall in a rapid effort to prevent a fainting patient from falling. In addition, the ventral and dorsal surfaces of both hands reflect silvery stab wounds where an abandoned red Doberman unsuccessfully tried to devour me when I worked in an airport animal shelter during my youth. Both of my hands appear as if I have dragged myself straight off a working farm or sailing ship like that of my ancestors, as the hands are adorned with thick knuckles, rough skin, and burly, wide fingers. Despite their lack of beauty, my hands work well and are strong and sturdy. I have been called "the Goddess with the Golden Hands" and "Brünhilde with the Iron Thumbs" with equal enthusiasm, and I am grateful for my gift.

~ ★ ~

The swelling just wouldn't go away. Delia's thumbs and knuckles were hopelessly inflamed and bent at the metacarpal-phalangeal joints in the classic sideswept pattern of rheumatoid arthritis. Interestingly, she had been referred to physical therapy not because of the arthritis, but for treatment of a small cyst located on the distal right index finger. The cyst was small, about the size of a pencil eraser, and although it was slightly painful, it was nothing in contrast to Delia's other hand problems. The cyst had manifested only recently and was unsightly rather than dysfunctional. It was located at the side of her distal interphalangeal (DIP) joint, but involved only the superficial dermal layers rather than the joint itself. Delia's main problem was the instability and inflammation attacking all of her other wrist, hand, thumb, and finger joints.

Delia's rheumatoid arthritis was old news but had recently worsened in both hands after she had to have surgery to replace one of her worn-out knees that had been destroyed by the same disease. Although the knee surgery had gone well, Delia was forced to use a front-wheeled walker to get around afterward; the increased pressure on her hands and also on her elbows from leaning on the walker was creating problems for her. Sadly, the stress and transient immobility of her knee surgery had also exacerbated her spinal stenosis, so it appeared that she was on the walker for good. "Aging isn't for sissies!" she reflected as we worked together on her puffy, twisted hands. I replied, "Yeah, I know . . . you're not alone in your thoughts. Just the other day I was driving along behind a pleasant-looking gray-haired gentleman, and as I drew closer to him I saw that he had a very nice gold license plate frame mounted on the back of his hunter green car. When I pulled up behind him at the next stoplight, I could see what he'd had engraved on the frame and had to laugh. There, in stark black letters, firmly etched into his lovely golden frame, was the sentiment, 'Screw the Golden Years'!" Delia laughed, saying that's exactly how she felt. "The only benefit to aging is that your eyesight starts to go," she said, her watery eyes sparkling with mirth. "I think that age-related visual loss is God's way of protecting you from seeing how you look as you get older."

Maintaining a sense of humor is essential, because aging brings an assortment of interconnected problems. Medications and therapeutic modalities or exercises designed to improve one of the patient's conditions may worsen another. For example, paraffin baths can provide a soothing form of deep heat to joints that aren't actively inflamed, but they may not be tolerated in patients with certain skin disorders. Cortisone injections to help directly reduce the inflammation of an affected joint or tendon may cause a dangerous spike in the blood sugars of a diabetic patient. The combined stressors of dovetailing diseases or repeated surgeries may bring on yet another condition, and this is what ended up happening to Delia.

Delia's hands and fingers had finally begun to improve, with the edema slowly waning, as she was able to start doing careful strengthening exercises to help stabilize her twisted, rickety hand and finger joints. Then, on a day when I hadn't expected to see her, Delia phoned. "You'll never believe it," she said, "but I have something new going on and I won't be able to see you for awhile . . . I have shingles! It's terribly painful, and the doctor wants me to stay home to try to recover. I don't know how long I've actually had it—you have had chicken pox before, haven't you?—because I might be contagious." I quickly assured Delia that I had indeed had chicken pox, and had in fact woken up on my eighth birthday in my little bed above the front door of my grandmother's house in England covered with the stuff.

I felt so sorry for Delia to have risen above so many obstacles with grace and spirit only to be knocked back down again on the eve of her improvement. But then I remembered what she used to tell me as we worked together: "I've had a great life, you know, and I can't complain. My dear husband and I traveled the world together and saw and experienced everything we wanted to . . . and now that he's gone, I hold my memories close to me and relive them when I see our son. I try to appreciate all the wonderful moments I've had, and realize how lucky I've been to really have experienced no problems at all with my health until I turned seventy-five! I can only wish the same for you."

I can only hope to bring some of Delia's vigor, spirit, and gratitude about life into my daily practice with future patients.

Part Four

The Lower Extremities

A wise man ought to realize that health is his most valuable possession.
—Hippocrates of Kos, Greek physician (460 BC–370 BC)

I have worked with thousands of patients in a multitude of different settings over the many years of my profession and have found a certain consistent truth. Across the board, the vast majority of patients who have experienced both upper and lower extremity injuries said that they preferred dealing with an incapacitated arm to having an injured leg. Our legs exist to carry us forward in life, and there is something fundamental to survival about being able to get about independently. Most patients agree that the very worst injury occurs when the right leg is involved, as this can significantly impact the ability to drive, curtailing freedom.

Our legs not only support our frames and enable us to move about at will, but over the time of generations have come to mean something more. When we give someone a leg up, we are physically helping them to get onto something such as a horse's back or are figuratively assisting them in some other way. If we pull someone's leg, we are usually teasing them about something as a shared joke. When we are left without a leg to stand on, we have metaphorically backed ourselves into a corner with no further way to factually support our position or excuse our poor behavior. Furthermore, "getting a leg over" refers to sexual intercourse, and this saying is sometimes coupled with the expression "legging it," which refers to the act of running away.

Shooting from the Hip

To celebrate life, you have to move your hips.
—*Trinidadian saying*

The hips are marvels of engineering. They provide the bridge between the spine (and all of its major attachments to the head and upper extremities) and the ground that we stand on. There is a delicate balance between the pull of the largest muscles in the body linking the hips to the pelvis and the sheer weight of our skeletons. Without hip joints, we would not be able to sit down nor would we be able to stand and walk smoothly, but instead would stiffly ambulate in a series of sideways, jerky, toppling motions.

The hip features prominently in our lives in a number of ways. We are considered "hip" if we are one of the in-crowd; we caution ourselves against the sins of overeating by telling each other "a moment on the lips, a lifetime on the hips"; we "shoot from the hip" when we speak bluntly and assertively; and we balance our babies and our saddles on our hips when we carry them around.

We tend to think of the hip as being the bony protuberance that marks the widest part of our lower extremity anatomy, but this is actually an outcropping of bone, the greater trochanter, which acts as an attachment point for many of the large hip and gluteal muscles. The ball and socket joint composed of the femoral head and the pelvic acetabulum is located much closer to the body's midline, and is designed to provide great stability as it transfers the forces incurred through ambulating, running, or leaping over rough ground. It is held in position by a tough fibrous joint capsule and a group of extremely strong ligaments, and is fed by several major arteries.

~ ★ ~

The patient had received his new hip the previous day and needed to learn how to use it. "Come on," said Pauline, my clinical rotation preceptor. "Bring Carlos over to the parallel bars so we can get him up on his feet." Earlier, we had helped Carlos transfer from his bed to the wheelchair in his hospital room without him actually bearing weight on the leg containing his new hip replacement, and he was now looking apprehensive.

It was the second week of my first-year PT clinical internship in a large acute care teaching hospital, and I was just beginning to become accustomed to the noisy, purposeful activity around the nursing station, the routine of securing the patient's chart as soon as the physician had flicked it shut, and the pervasive hospital smells that lingered on my clothing long after I had reached home. This patient was "mine"—and as a special treat, I had been allowed to observe his total hip replacement surgery in the operating room, watching cautiously over the orthopedic surgeon's shoulder. I had been incredibly nervous in the operating theater, even though I was careful to look away at the moment the surgeon made the initial incision into the patient's hip. Although I have never been particularly squeamish about blood, during my first year of undergraduate science I had watched an ovarian transfer technique being performed on a white laboratory rabbit and remember being bewildered by the sudden buzzing noises in my ears and whirling black spots in front of my eyes. As I dully realized that I was on the brink of passing out, I had abruptly sat down and stuck my head between my knees. Despite my efforts to desensitize myself, I have yet to conquer this reaction to the first incision, even when performed on the inert bodies in the cadaver lab. Once the first cut is made and I can see the underlying muscle and bone, I'm fine—at that point, it all simply becomes anatomy, rather than an actual person or animal being violated.

When Pauline and I knocked on the door of Carlos's room to collect him for his physical therapy session, I realized I had not yet officially met him or even seen his face; the previous day every part of him except his right hip had been swathed in surgical drapes. I whispered to Pauline, "Isn't he too young for a hip replacement?" She reminded me that his preoperative diagnosis was hip avascular necrosis (AVN), a condition in which the ball of the head of the femur loses its blood supply and dies. Although there are many causes of AVN, it primarily occurs secondary to trauma, alcohol abuse, or steroid use, and is common in young men under the age of fifty. Fortunately, it turned out that my patient Carlos was young and slim, and he would surely have no trouble lifting himself out of the wheelchair and standing up in the parallel bars in the hospital's basement to take his first steps. The only complication was that he spoke no English, so we communicated with each other through our rudimentary hospital Spanish and a combination of vigorous hand gestures.

We had coordinated our therapy session with the nursing staff to correspond with Carlos's pain medications, and were prepared for a fairly routine session. I had practiced transfer techniques at PT school and knew that even the freshest postsurgical total hip patient could safely put his full weight on the leg without damaging the surgical implant. I smiled at Carlos and gestured that I would place a gait belt around his midsection to give me a handhold on his waist for safety. He smiled weakly back at me and nodded his acquiescence, but seemed a bit sweaty and clammy as I secured the belt into place around his blue patterned hospital gown and robe. "Okay, Pauline, we're all set," I said as I moved the wheelchair between the bars in preparation for Carlos's standing debut. Pauline stepped in front of Carlos to move his footrests out of the way, and said, "See one, do one, teach one . . . I'll help him up the first time, then you can have a try. Just follow behind him with the chair as he walks down the bars, so he won't have to turn around to sit." I glanced down at the wheelchair brakes to be sure they were on, and checked that the hose of the Foley catheter bag collecting Carlos's urine was free of the wheels. Carlos moaned a little, but Pauline smiled at him sympathetically and said, "Levántase, por favor!" as she moved her hands upward.

Pauline carefully gripped his gait belt and was watching to be sure he kept the right leg sufficiently forward so as not to allow his right hip to bend beyond 90 degrees to guard against dislocation, when I noticed fresh sweat appear at the collar of his robe. I said, "Pauline, wait, I think he—" She looked up right as poor Carlos convulsed, releasing a fragrant stream of projectile vomit directly into her face. We both gagged along with Carlos but mercifully added no additional vomit to the spreading pool at Pauline's feet. I rushed to grab a stack of towels to sponge off Carlos and Pauline, and felt guiltily grateful I had been behind the chair at the time.

Especially in the acute care setting, treatment often requires that therapists manage a bewildering array of devices, tubes, belts, and rules. But regardless of these necessary distractions, I learned a vivid, valuable lesson that day—it is important that PTs keep their full attention on the patient at all times.

~ ★ ~

I had always associated hip bursitis with the elderly until I developed a painful case of it during my early twenties. I had been a longtime advocate of sleeping on hard surfaces and had enjoyed using my thin, flat futon without any problems for many years. Like most people, I had a favorite side upon which I slept; in my case, the left side was the best because it allowed me to look out of the window while lying in bed, with my jet-black feline companion, Calamity, nestled in behind my legs. Gradually, I noticed that my left hip would start to burn within a scant thirty seconds after I turned into my favorite position, and I lost night after night of sleep as I tossed and turned in my quest to find a comfortable spot. I would feel fine if I rested my weight either a little bit in front of or behind my greater trochanter (the lateral prominence at the upper part of the femur), but I just couldn't lie squarely on the outside of the hip itself.

Years later, I realized that the cause of the problem was my greater trochanteric bursa. The bursa's role is to pad the overlying muscles and tendons, preventing them from rubbing against the underlying bone, so that movement is smooth and painless. Once the bursa becomes inflamed, however, it becomes increasingly aggravated by the movement of the soft tissues repeatedly sliding across it, creating a vicious cycle of pain. Bursitis can be caused by direct compression such as occurs with lying on the bursa or even falling on it, the results of which I remember seeing in one of my PT school classmates. In a former life, Catherine had been a junior ice skating champion to the point of competing at national level, and over the years she had sustained innumerable falls onto the ice. Since she usually ended up slamming onto one of her hips, they took the brunt of each fall on the hard, frozen surface. I recall the day in PT school when we were discussing hip problems and Catherine pulled up the hem of her shorts. Aghast, I could see that instead of the normal convex hourglass-like contours of the outer hip, Catherine sported large indentations where her hip bursae used to be. All of those icy falls had resulted in inflammation and then eventual necrosis and permanent damage of the hip bursae and surrounding soft tissues.

Hip bursitis can also be caused by repetitive movements such as those used for hiking or cycling, when the iliotibial band repeatedly swishes across the bursa thousands of times within a brief period. In addition, when muscles are short and tight following traumatic injury or surgery, the bursa beneath the soft tissues can become compressed and subsequently inflamed. When this happens, the bursa can protrude (something no girl wants to have happen to her hip!) and is exquisitely painful to touch.

The solution to my problem was to quit aggravating the left hip bursa with compression from my hard futon, and to stretch out the relatively tighter muscles in my left leg to reduce the repetitive friction. Because of my longtime habit of "hanging out" on my left leg most of the time, the left quadriceps muscles and iliotibial band were noticeably tighter than those of my right leg. This was probably because my poor left leg had to work much harder than the right one throughout the course of the day, and after awhile the muscles simply learned to become hypervigilant and primed to contract, slowly tightening up without my noticing.

The left leg tightness problem had been briskly accelerated shortly after I had acquired Atlas. At some point during his early years, Atlas had been chased, whipped, and hissed at by someone standing on his right side. I figured this out because he was nervous about unfamiliar sounds coming from his off side, and was jumpy and panicky if anyone or anything approached him from the right. I was progressively working with him to regain his trust, but he had not yet conquered his fear on the day of the accident.

I had been schooling Atlas in the arena one early morning before heading off to the clinic, working on his flexibility with left-handed circles (he was much more pliant to the right, probably because he would habitually lie on his left side with his spine curled in right side bend and his legs tucked up to the right), when the neighbor's sprinklers turned on with a hiss to our right. Poor Atlas completely lost it and bolted away for all he was worth to escape the anticipated pain, oblivious to my spirited attempts to stop him. We quickly ran out of room as he raced in a blind panic to the far side of the arena. What was I to do? He couldn't stop in time, so was he going to jump the fence or crash through it? I grimly held on, thinking only of his safety and how to divert him from his crash course, when at the eleventh hour he swerved at a full speed gallop, depositing me into the arena fence with my left lateral thigh crushed against the fence post. Although Atlas was safe, I was in agony.

I was able to heave myself up to calm a shaken Atlas and put him away, and brokenly limped off to work. As the day wore on, I found that I was less and less able to bear weight on my left leg. Could I have sustained a hairline fracture that was widening? The pain was becoming excruciating. As soon as I had finished with patient care, I took myself off to the closest doctor's office for an X-ray. The good news was that I didn't have a femoral fracture. The bad news was that I had crushed my lateral femoral cutaneous nerve, and it was quite upset. Compression of the lateral femoral cutaneous nerve, also known as meralgia paresthetica, can be caused not only by direct trauma but also from entrapment anywhere along the sensory nerve's path, whether at its origin at L2 and L3, along the inguinal ligament, through the psoas muscle, or at its destination in the anterolateral thigh. Corticosteroids to calm the hypersensitive nerve, a stretching program, and time all served to eventually solve my problem, but I was left with a shortened left vastus lateralis muscle that contributed to my general tightness and long-standing bursal irritability.

The cure may be simple, but isn't always easy—as I resumed my stretching program with increased vigor, the bursa became freshly irritated. I discovered later that this is a common reaction, because in the course of stretching the tight muscles overlying the greater trochanter, the bursa becomes transiently more compressed and inflamed. The key is to stick with it, a true "no pain no gain" situation. Ultimately, Calamity and I were able to return to our favorite sleeping position, although my left greater trochanteric bursa remains sensitive to prolonged pressure. On such days, I feel elderly but use the painful reminder as a cue to get back into my stretching program to help me remain fit for life.

~ ★ ~

A fair number of subacute care hospital patients who must spend time at geriatric rehabilitation centers are widows and widowers who have broken their hips and are subsequently recovering from surgery. Despite the fact that most of them would prefer to go directly home after a brief stay at the acute care hospital, the sad reality is that with a departed spouse and often no family living nearby, they need more help to get back on their feet before safely returning home again. Of all types of patients these are my favorites, for they remind me of my own beloved grandparents and I am eager to help them regain their independence and dignity.

Stella was one such patient. She had been living alone in the family home for nearly ten years after her husband had died, with only her little black cat, Tommy, to keep her company. Unhappily, one day Tommy became mixed up in Stella's legs as she came downstairs to fix their breakfasts, and she ended up on the floor with a broken hip. Stella was a gentle, petite woman with only one desire—to return home to her darling Tommy. For now, her kind neighbor was looking after Tommy each day, but Stella still had some healing to do before she could go home to look after herself and her little cat.

For several reasons, the surgeons had decided to pin Stella's hip via an open reduction internal fixation (ORIF) surgery instead of giving her a total hip replacement. Despite her advanced age and small stature, Stella did not have significant osteoporosis and was thought to have strong enough bone to "take" the stabilizing metal plate and screws well—osteoporotic bone tends to collapse when drilled into. In addition, Stella had just cracked the femoral neck, or the portion of the bone that bridges the gap between the hip joint and the rest of the femur, leaving the ball and socket hip joint intact and producing no fragment displacement. Stella was also mentally sharp, and would be able to comply with the postsurgical regimen of partial weight bearing until the fracture had begun to mend; patients who aren't able to follow directions or who have dementia don't understand that they shouldn't put all their weight on the operated leg, and will suffer from bones that refuse to heal.

Thus, Stella ended up staying for a short while at the geriatric rehabilitation hospital where I worked. Although she was less than enthusiastic about this prospect, she was eager to do whatever she could in her efforts to try to get home sooner. It was my job to help her regain her independent ambulatory status, make sure she remained safe with her weight-bearing status, and to rebuild her endurance in conjunction with the OTs so that Stella could manage on her own again. I saw Stella twice each day to guide her through the necessary strengthening exercises and activities to restore her ability to move in bed, transfer from her bed into a chair, and walk with safety, all while keeping her balance and maintaining partial weight bearing on the operated leg.

Part of providing therapy to patients in the rehabilitation unit of a geriatric convalescent hospital is to help them relearn the mechanics of getting about after surgery during the most mundane tasks. For Stella, this meant receiving instruction on how to maneuver her stiff, freshly repaired leg into clothing and around her walker; how to take a shower and put on her shoes; and how to manage in the bathroom. Physical and occupational therapists alike worked with Stella to help her learn how to balance as she brushed her teeth and made her bed. One afternoon I went to collect Stella in order to bring her to the therapy room so we could work on balance exercises and ambulation. I found her reclining on the bed, having taken a rest after lunch. Stella was willing enough to come along for her therapy session, but first said that she needed to use the restroom. She had been ringing her call bell for at least ten minutes, but no nurse had come along to answer it and help her to the toilet. No problem, I said—this was all part of the therapy day—so I assisted her out of bed to walk the few feet to the restroom using her walker, making sure that she kept balanced but without too much weight on the operated leg. I had a firm hold on her gait belt, the canvas belt we routinely looped around each patient's waist as a handhold for safety, and encouraged her to traverse the distance carefully. Stella made it into the bathroom without further ado, and after she was comfortably seated I placed the bathroom call bell in her hand and stepped outside to give her privacy.

After a few minutes, Stella called out to me to indicate she was finished and needed some help. Fortunately, she was pretty nimble and had successfully wiped herself and generally tidied up, but as she still tended to pull herself up from seats using the walker, she needed someone nearby so as not to lose her balance backward. I knocked and entered to find her poised to stand up, her long anti-embolism stockings and underwear wreathed around her ankles. I reminded her that it was acceptable to stand on both legs with equal pressure since she was restricted to 50 percent weight bearing (when standing with the weight squarely on both feet, the weight is spread out fifty-fifty), but asked her to push up from the raised toilet seat handles and nearby grab bar instead of the walker. I took hold of her gait belt, and Stella stood and arranged her clothing without incident. I was at her side, ready to guide her out of the room and down the hallway to the therapy room, but she resisted. Perplexed, I asked what the matter was. Firmly, Stella announced, "I want to inspect my stool." I didn't like to ask why, so merely helped her maneuver the walker around in the tiny bathroom so that she could peer into the toilet bowl. After a long moment, she declared herself satisfied and permitted me to guide her out of the restroom. I reached back to activate the toilet flush, mystified.

We reached the treatment room with Stella keeping a beautiful partial weight-bearing pattern on the affected leg, and after a brief rest she turned to me and explained why she was so interested in the contents of her toilet. She had suffered from constipation-based irritable bowel syndrome for some time, and had recently also begun to experience anemia. The doctors planned to perform a series of tests to see if they could determine the cause of her anemia once she had recovered from her hip surgery, including a colonoscopy and an upper and lower gastrointestinal series. Until then, she was determined to keep watch over the results in the toilet bowl so that she could accurately report the presence of blood. Mystery solved.

In the therapy room, I had Stella practice keeping the right amount of weight over her injured leg as she moved by asking her to shift her weight on and off a common bathroom scale. We worked on activities to improve her balance by attempting a partial weight-bearing version of the drunk driving test, in which the participant must stand with one foot in front of the other (the tandem Romberg test), and batted balloons back and forth to each other as Stella stood near a railing for safety, the wheelchair behind her "just in case." Stella maintained a cheerful disposition throughout all of the silly exercises I could throw at her and chatted to me all the while about Tommy, her primary source of inspiration.

After our session together, we returned to her room and Stella conspiratorially asked me to bring her purse over to her. I did so, and watched patiently as she rummaged through it for a small, worn folder. Her face lighting up, she pulled a photograph of Tommy out of the battered folder for me to admire with a trembling hand. There before me was a picture of the mangiest looking black tomcat I had ever seen in my life. He looked thin and old, with one of his ears missing some fur and a few of his whiskers turned white. I looked at the frail old cat, and turned to Stella with my heart bursting with compassion. "Isn't he beautiful?" she sighed as she gazed at Tommy's picture adoringly. I remembered my own dearly loved cat-friend Calamity, who I had lost to kidney failure a few years previously. She had been the light of my life and a constant friend and companion for sixteen years, seeing me through many rites of passage, including first leaving home, graduating from PT school, and entering into marriage. In Calamity's old age she had also begun to look tattered and faded, but I had never noticed—I only saw her with the eyes of love. "He's gorgeous," I gently agreed.

Everyone needs a reason to live, whether during rehabilitation from injury or simply when getting out of bed every morning. For some, motivation takes the form of competing with a hospital roommate or with themselves to achieve a "personal best." But for others, the desire to get better is fueled by their attachments to loved ones, whether human or otherwise—the importance of such relationships mustn't be overlooked as a strong motivating factor that enhances patient compliance and ensures successful recovery.

~ ★ ~

Our receptionist and Jill-of-all-trades sidled up to me in the narrow hallway of our outpatient clinic and murmured into my right ear, "Watch out for this one—she seems pretty tense." Intrigued, I proceeded to the second treatment room clutching my new patient's chart. All I knew was that Joy was here for assessment of her back, buttock, hip, and knee pain. At least she had arrived on time, so I had the full thirty minutes to assess nearly half of her body. When I knocked and entered the room, I was confronted with a very petite Asian lady in her early seventies. Joy was impeccably dressed in a coordinated pantsuit outfit of different shades of green. Her makeup was expertly applied, and each hair was beautifully styled into place. The only part that didn't match was her pair of black patent leather shoes, which were incredibly scuffed and worn. She smiled nervously as I greeted her, but seemed normal enough.

In the course of my assessment I discovered that her biggest problem area was in her hips. Her joint range of motion was incredibly restricted and her leg muscles were extremely weak, the right worse than the left. Then I asked her to walk. Poor Joy shuffled along with baby steps, her weight precariously balanced on the lateral borders and balls of her feet as she swayed unsteadily down the hallway. I was amazed that she had driven herself to the clinic and climbed the stairs (the elevator was an option for our less mobile patients, but Joy had confessed to a longtime claustrophobia and had shunned elevators for years). "I can't help it, but I walk like a duck!" she exclaimed as she shakily navigated her way back into the treatment room. "Either a duck, or one of those ancient Chinese ladies with bound feet—it takes me forever to get anywhere. I also have so much pain in my right leg when I try to stand up after sitting for awhile, it feels like ten out of ten pain," she said. "I even have to keep wearing these same shoes because they're so light and they slip on . . . I can't bend down to tie a lace or fasten a buckle. I can't even reach to wash my feet! Can you do anything to help me?" she asked.

After a thorough evaluation, I began treating her by gently stretching and massaging her tight hip and buttock muscles, knowing that with her muscles cramped into such a short, disadvantaged position, she would be unable to use them properly. She was unable to lie on her stomach for me to access her hips, so we compromised with her lying first on one hip and then the other, her legs well supported on pillows, as she was too stiff with arthritis and muscle contractures to bring her knees together. As always, when I begin to place my hands on someone I explain what I am going to do and why; but then, Joy interrupted me with her own story.

"This is why I specifically requested a woman," she said. "When I went to see Dr. D, the nurse checked me out first and said that since the doctor would be mostly looking at my legs, there was no need to change into a gown. So, after the nurse took my blood pressure and wrote down my weight I just sat there waiting. But, instead of Dr. D, some guy came into the room, walked up to me, and asked me to stand . . . then when I did, he pulled down my pants!" Joy giggled nervously, her hand covering her face in remembered humiliation. "I was so embarrassed! He even was looking 'in the front,' which didn't seem right . . . I wondered if he was trying to get a cheap thrill, you know, such a young man and everything. It turns out he was the doctor in training, but I still feel ashamed."

"Did you tell Dr. D what happened?" I asked.

"No, I didn't. Do you think I should?" she replied.

"Yes!" I answered. "I know it's a teaching hospital, but that resident is there to learn about all aspects of patient care, not just perform clinical tests. There is a whole common courtesy and respect issue that all health professionals need to remember—that their patients aren't just a sore hip or leg, but a whole person with needs and wants and feelings. Do you think he would've walked up to his own mother and pulled down her pants? No, of course not! When you go back to see Dr. D next week, tell her what happened so she can help this cavalier young guy learn something."

My feelings of outrage on Joy's behalf calmed as I worked on her tight hips, and our conversation lapsed into more neutral territory. But, as I thought about Joy's experience later, I became freshly agitated and felt like rushing over to the hospital to de-pants the brash young doctor as a lesson—how would he feel? In the process of learning, health professionals can become abrupt; when we focus so intently on locating the diagnosis, we sometimes forget about the patient's sensibilities. At the other extreme, very experienced doctors and therapists can become jaded and neglectful of yet one more patient's hip problem. I find it helpful to remember the Golden Rule—treat others as you would wish to be treated—but, for those times that I feel rushed or agitated, I tweak the rule a little and think instead about treating others as I would like my favorite family members to be treated. This helps me stay on track.

~ ★ ~

Total hip replacements can be tricky, and they require great skill on the part of the surgeon. Many factors go into a successful outcome, which depends upon the healing abilities of the patient, the type of prosthetic replacement chosen, the patient's age, and the ability to comply with movement restrictions following surgery. Traditionally in the United States, most hip replacements were performed with a posterior approach, requiring the surgeon to cut through layers of gluteal muscles and the posterior joint capsule to reach the damaged or broken joint. Now, the mini-incision is revolutionizing hip replacements by reducing trauma to the patient and creating a faster recovery. Some surgeons are now incorporating an anterior approach to the hip by making an incision in the front of the hip then carefully dissecting down past the femoral artery and nerves to reach the hip joint; this approach significantly reduces the risk of dislocation, an ever-present postsurgical problem. However, the anterior approach requires extra skill and practice; you want to be sure to choose a surgeon who has done more than ten before he turns his scalpel on you.

Most surgeons advise their patients with severe degenerative hip osteoarthritis that "they'll know" when the time is right to go ahead with the operation. But even if the preoperative bone measurements are accurate, the prosthesis is the right size and arrives at the surgical suite at the correct time, and the surgery goes well, the new hip still won't last forever. With time, the prosthesis eventually degrades and loosens as tiny fragments of metal, plastic, or ceramic release into the surrounding bone.

Willard had been coming into the clinic for some time for an old back injury. He was a veteran of a head-on car collision, complete with a pelvic fracture in his youth; several spinal surgeries to decompress various spinal nerve roots and help him walk again without foot drop; and an earlier total hip replacement. We had become friends during one of his outpatient spinal surgery rehabs, and I had enjoyed helping Willard return to his former regimen of slowly bicycling around the neighborhood and doing the family shopping. However, I noticed that despite improvements in his spinal muscle tone and trunk control, Willard continued to walk with a slight limp that necessitated the use of a cane.

"It's a good thing I have the body of a ditch digger," Willard said contentedly as I released his tight back muscles and encouraged him to exercise his weak leg. "I'm sure that most ordinary people wouldn't have done nearly as well as I have after all these injuries. I don't really need this cane for anything but my balance; see—I barely press on it at all." I took a closer look at him, and asked him to try walking without the cane. Since canes can offset as much as 50 percent of the body's weight away from the injured side, I was curious to see how much Willard really did rely on his cane. Sure enough, Willard developed a distinct twist and side-bobbing lateral motion as he bore weight on the left leg—the classic Trendelenberg gait pattern. This pattern is indicative of weakness in the hip abductors, especially the gluteus medius muscle, and is frequently seen with hip trouble. I felt a frisson of fear.

"How long ago was your hip surgery?" I asked.

"About eight years ago . . . why?" Willard responded.

"When was your last follow-up X-ray?"

"I don't remember. Maybe about three or four years ago?"

"You might want to make an appointment with your hip surgeon." I urged. "It's hard to tell when there's overlapping pathology like you have with long-term back and leg weakness from all those previous injuries, but it looks to me like your hip is a big part of the problem, and you might just want to rule it out."

Two weeks passed before Willard finally showed up again on my schedule. He was now using a cane in each hand, and had news to report. "My orthopedist says that my artificial hip socket has worn out and has been pushed up into my pelvis by over an inch! It's unstable and I'm scheduled for a revision surgery with a specialist right around Thanksgiving . . . until then, he wants me to use crutches or a walker to keep the weight off it. Do I have to use a walker? I'm really much more comfortable with my canes."

I slowly said, "I think that you should follow your surgeon's advice with this one. Why not use the walker just until you have surgery? I think that you should limit the damage as best as you can, and you might be able to keep more weight off the hip using the walker for a week or two."

Willard's home life was busy, with Willard acting as the primary caregiver for his wife, who had severe emphysema. Despite needing a constant flow of oxygen and having such poor endurance that she hadn't left the house in more than three years, his wife was a smoker who wasn't able to catch her breath long enough to help out around the house. So, after Willard's delicate surgery for a pelvic bone graft and new hip socket, he had to enter a convalescent hospital until he could properly get back up on his feet. A few days after his surgery, I went to visit him in a skilled nursing facility where I had formerly worked. All the faces at the facility were new, as none of the staff from my day had stayed on. I dutifully signed in at the front desk and made my way down the familiar scrubbed hallways. As always, there was a smell redolent of overcooked hospital food, an assortment of long-term care residents sadly trolling the hallways for company in their wheelchairs, and an aloof nursing staff.

I found my way to Willard's room, knocked, and entered. The first bed was empty, the patient gazing at me suspiciously from his vantage point in an olive green vinyl chair near the doorway. I smiled at him and indicated my desire to see his roommate. He stared at me uncomprehendingly, so I persisted in my path toward the window. Sure enough, there, surrounded by a frothing sea of rumpled sheets, lay my friend Willard. He looked small and frail, with large, dark circles beneath his eyes and extreme pallor upon his skin. He too, stared at me vacantly. Then his expression cleared. "Anne! It's so good to see you. I just got back into bed before lunch for a rest, and here you are." Willard reached out to me, so I stepped into his thin, bruised arms and kissed his unshaven cheek. He immediately whipped aside the covers to expose the neat line of staples holding the skin of his left hip together; the surgeon had gone back in using the old posterior scar as a guide. "It looks good," I said as I surveyed his dry, filleted white leg. "How did everything go?"

"Well, the doc says I'm a high risk for dislocating my artificial hip since this was my second surgery on it and I had dislocation problems after the first one . . . he wants me to wear a cast-brace on my hip for awhile to help keep it in place. Frankly, I take it off every chance I get! You know me; I'm fine if I just put a sheet between my knees to keep my skin from sticking together when I lie on my side—I like to sleep nude, you know—and then I don't have any problems."

"Ah, Willard . . . you know, you really shouldn't do that right now! The naked part is fine if you feel too hot, but if your knees come close together you're really increasing the risk of your hip dislocating! Promise me you'll use the brace, or at least an abduction pillow, for awhile. I don't want you to have any more setbacks!"

Willard assented with good grace, and changed the subject to ask about my horses. He had always been interested in the horses because of his farming background and the fact that his daughter raised horses, so I filled him in on my sad news. My much-loved old Irish horse, Riley, had suddenly died. After a long jumping career, followed by a happy semi-retirement as a trail horse, Riley had become increasingly fragile during the preceding few months and had begun to have difficulty rising from the ground after having a good roll in the dirt to scratch his back. A couple of times I'd had to boost him up, but he had been enjoying life and reveling in his "top horse" status at the barn, and had learned not to get down and roll unless I was there. Then one early morning at work I received the dreaded phone call—"your horse is dying"—Riley was down and struggling. I dropped everything, assigning some understanding patients to another therapist and canceling the rest, and raced out to the stables as I frantically phoned my veterinarian from the car. When I reached Riley, I could see that this was it, the definitive moment when I knew he was ready to go. He was shaking, dizzy, and confused. My compassionate vet, Gary, helped me understand through my tears that Riley had probably had a stroke, and although we could try to help him get back up on his feet, there were no guarantees for his recovery. I could see that it wouldn't be kind to try, and asked Gary to call my husband for me while I stroked Riley's noble head and calmed him with reassuring words of love. Riley quieted a little, and when my husband joined us we said good-bye and held him in our arms as Gary slipped the needle into Riley's neck. This was one of the worst days of my life, but I could finally understand Tennyson's words "'Tis better to have loved and lost, than never to have loved at all." Riley had been my kindred spirit, friend, and partner for more than twenty years and had died at the ripe old age of thirty-one. I was lucky to have had him for so long and remain grateful that I could ease his passing.

Although I had gone to visit Willard to lift his spirits after a long and complicated surgery, he had done a lot for me in return by sympathetically listening to my story. Sometimes, the exchange of personal information between the patient and therapist goes two ways, and healing can be mutual.

The Controlling Knee

A woman is as young as her knees.

—Mary Quant, English fashion designer and miniskirt inventor (1934–)

The knees represent our willingness to move forward in life. They serve as a mirror for our ability to bend gracefully as we adapt to daily stresses, and reflect our aptitude for mental and physical flexibility. The knee is the largest joint in the body and the main weight-bearing joint of the lower extremity. However, despite its stability, it is frequently vulnerable to injury—knee problems are the most common cause of visits to the doctor each year.

The knee works as a hinge joint to bend and straighten over an enormous range of motion, encompassing up to 160 degrees of flexion. Despite a small amount of rotational glide, the knee should bend only in one plane, a feat made possible by the strong ligaments around and within the joint that act as support straps. The medial and lateral collateral ligaments help keep the knee safe from being sideswiped, and the anterior and posterior cruciate ligaments cross each other deep within the joint to prevent excessive rotation and anterior or posterior translation of the tibia against the femur. The bony surfaces of the knee joint are further stabilized and cushioned by inner and outer crescent-shaped cartilaginous cushions known as the medial and lateral meniscus. The ends of the femur and tibia are also capped by cartilage to ensure friction-free gliding with every step we take, although aging, trauma, arthritis, or disease can eventually destroy this protective layer of padding and result in the need for a knee replacement.

Horses can sleep standing up due to their ability to relax onto the ligaments supporting their knee joints, which are actually located in the horse's anterior hip area, also known as the stifle. To accomplish this, they activate part of the quadriceps, the vastus medialis obliquus (VMO) muscle, to actively stabilize the patella, enabling them to stand with little effort. The human patella is similarly controlled by the VMO muscle, which helps to coordinate smooth patellar gliding within the femoral groove located at the distal femur with every step we take. Knee control is accomplished by the harmonious co-contraction of the quadriceps and hamstrings muscles, and any deviation from strong, flexible muscles can result in injury.

~ ★ ~

Steven was an active young man in his late twenties who arrived at the clinic brandishing a prescription for help with patellofemoral pain syndrome. This condition is one in which the patella will laterally slide out of control within the femoral groove, and is often caused by a combination of tight outer leg muscles (iliotibial band and lateral quadriceps) and weakness of the VMO portion of the inner quadriceps. This muscular imbalance creates an asymmetrical pull on the patella, which typically drags it to the outside of the femoral groove, creating friction and wearing down the underlying cartilage. The usually vague, global pain is normally felt at the front of the knee underneath the patella, and becomes worse with concussive movements caused by activities such as running, jumping, and hiking down hills. Although I had been held up for ten minutes with my previous patient, I entered the room with a smile and reached out to shake Steven's hand, saying, "Sorry to keep you waiting. It's nice to meet you, Steven—my name is Anne. Do you go by Steven, or Steve?"

"I go by Steven . . . and it's spelled the right way, with a 'v.'"

Ah, yes—one of those. I asked Steven with a "v" how long he'd had knee pain, what the aggravating factors were, and where he usually felt the pain. After obtaining a fairly unremarkable history, I invited him to show me his sore knee. Steven stood up rapidly, and in one seamless motion dropped his pants to the floor. Fortunately, he was wearing underwear beneath his khakis, but his boxer shorts were gapping rudely to reveal a gratuitous, untidy forest. I gave no visible response, but merely asked him to step over to the treatment table so we could take a proper look at his knee injury. Steven dragged up his pants, hopped onto the treatment table, and proceeded to draw his pant leg up to expose his knee from below. I dryly commented that this was a much easier way to examine the knee, and continued my assessment with his personal areas more discreetly covered. From that point on, he behaved himself. (There are always patients who try to push the limits of propriety. Many of them are smart-aleck young men trying to get a reaction; others are simply ignorant of the finer social niceties. Unless I feel physically threatened, I strive to maintain my professional demeanor and ignore the incident so as not give the offender the satisfaction of a shocked response).

After testing Steven's strength, muscular tightness, and joint range of motion, I placed my hands upon his leg. Flexibility testing had revealed a very tight right iliotibial (IT) band, which is the connective tissue strap that runs from the hip to the knee along the outside of the leg. A shortened IT band can be a major contributor to patellar instability and lateral tracking out of the femoral groove. With palpation I could feel and see that Steven's right patella had shifted toward the outside of the knee, with the lateral edge actually hanging over the cliff of the femoral condyle. In this ill-fated position, the patella would be forced to glide up and down along the sharp crest of the joint's edge rather than cruise smoothly within the natural U-shaped depression in which it was intended to reside. Poor patellar alignment can be improved by stretching out the tight IT band with massage and sliding it across a foam roller, like using a rolling pin on bread dough; by enhancing the strength of the VMO portion of the quadriceps muscle to pull the inner patella medially; and by training the patella to glide in the correct position while holding it in place with special tape (the McConnell taping technique). I tend to use a combination of all of these approaches to alleviate the pain and restore normal joint mechanics as quickly as possible; in this way, the damage to the underlying cartilage is minimized.

I explained the problem and my proposed treatment plan to Steven, who gave me his consent to begin deep tissue mobilization on his IT band in order to increase the tissue extensibility and to stretch it. I made sure he was comfortably ensconced on the treatment table sitting with a supportive pillow behind his low back and a towel roll beneath his knee to stabilize it, and began. At first I used the pads of all my fingers welded together in unison to familiarize him with my touch, and then I pulled out the big guns—my thumbs. My thumbs probably should be registered as lethal weapons: they are quite stiff, with very little give in them; this stiffness enables me to generate significant pressure and allows me to easily reach the deep tissues of the body. I started lightly and then progressed along the distal IT band with increasing pressure, chatting lightly to Steven about his job.

"What is it you do for a living, Steven?" I asked as I pushed against his right lateral knee and distal IT band.

"Wow, that's pretty sore!" he responded. "I'm actually a helicopter pilot, which is a pretty fun way to make money. I also like . . ."

Dead silence. I glanced up at Steven's face, only to realize that he was passing out. His eyelids were fluttering and his upper body was falling away from me, his head rapidly approaching the wall. Quickly, I leaped up from my stool and grabbed his right shoulder to save his head and center his now unconscious form on the treatment table before pulling the lever to lower the backrest into a flat position. I looked at him again—he was out cold. I pulled the pillow up behind his head and was just considering leaving the room to call for help when his eyelids began to flutter again. Steven woke up with a comical expression of confusion on his face. "What happened?" he said as his eyes finally focused on mine.

"Well, you passed out," I said with a small smile. "Sometimes it happens in response to pain or after surgery, when the body is still adjusting to life after being cut on. Do you want some water?"

"No . . . I can't believe I passed out! How long was I out? That's never happened before. Can I ask you something?"

"Ask away."

"Can we just keep this between ourselves? I'll never live it down if the guys find out about this . . . and hey, I'm sorry about earlier."

I affected not to know what he was referring to, and returned to my deep tissue mobilization, albeit with a lighter pressure.

~ ★ ~

Some patients exhibit more stoicism, or what my husband refers to as "intestinal fortitude," than others. One of the most self-controlled people that I know and emulate is my own mother. She has had many injuries and surgeries over her lifetime, but manages to sail through some of the toughest procedures with a level head and robust demeanor without turning a hair. She had undergone one knee replacement surgery before I had become a PT, and amazed me with her rapid recovery and apparent indifference to pain. I could only appreciate what a truly remarkable feat this was when I scrubbed in to observe a patient's knee replacement surgery many years later. The surgeons were artisans and carpenters, wielding bone saws, jigs, and Dremel tools with flair and panache as they removed sections of the patient's leg in two places before hammering on the new prosthesis. A knee replacement is one of the most painful surgeries a patient can endure, and it is truly miraculous that patients can stand up and walk on a freshly replaced joint within hours of such a necessarily brutal surgery.

When the time came for my mother to undergo an arthroscopy to remove torn cartilage (partial meniscectomy) from her other knee, we both thought that it would be a walk in the park compared to most of her other surgeries. The arthroscopic surgery was intended to shave the back of my mother's patella to smooth the roughened surfaces and to remove the cartilage fragments, or "loose mice" inside the joint, that had broken off when she had torn her medial meniscus with a fall. I went with her to the same-day surgery center, and settled down with my computer to work on a continuing education course while I waited. The surgeon, a gruff but experienced curmudgeon, had assured me that the surgery would be over so fast that I wouldn't even have time to eat a sandwich, let alone develop a new course. So, I became increasingly anxious as the minutes and then the hours ticked past.

Finally after more than two hours had elapsed, the surgeon poked his head out into the waiting room. "There were complications," he explained. "The surgery itself went fine, but the anesthesia team had trouble getting your Mom stable and we're going to have to keep her here overnight. Why don't you come on back and see her now?"

I swiftly bundled my computer back into its bag and followed him into the recovery room. He melted away, and I was left facing a very anxious-looking nurse hovering over my mother's gurney. "What on earth happened?" I asked, meaning, "What the hell have you done to her?!" The nurse nervously straightened the stethoscope slung around her neck, and said, "The anesthesia team had a lot of trouble getting her intubated, and once they got the tube in, they realized that it was actually in her stomach, not her lungs. Unfortunately, by this time your Mom wasn't breathing and was getting pretty deoxygenated, so they had to call the team from the emergency room over to help them get the tube in the right place. I'm sorry to say that in the process, your Mom's front teeth got broken and her lungs have collapsed. We'll have to transport her across the street to the main hospital to keep her on oxygen and monitor her overnight."

I was incredulous. I had never heard of a simple knee arthroscopy going quite so wrong and hoped that she hadn't suffered any brain damage. I went over to her bedside, took her hand, and called her name softly. She was so pale, and all of her hair curiously seemed to have turned gray. She opened her eyes and stared at me with confusion that slowly dawned into recognition. Thank goodness, she knew me. But all of my experience in hospitals and clinics counted for nothing. I felt so helpless—years of PT practice had given me the confidence to assist thousands of patients in all sorts of ways, but the scene unfolding in front of me was beyond my ability to cope. The nurse anxiously intervened, saying, "We'll have to transport her over to the main hospital in a wheelchair, but I don't think I can transfer her off the gurney on my own. I was just going to call for a couple of orderlies to help."

I said, "Never mind—I can do it! I think you've done enough."

This, I could handle. Transfers are life's blood to therapists, who can move patients back and forth between all kinds of surfaces without batting an eye. I gently bent over my mother's still form, and asked her if she thought she could get into the adjacent wheelchair with my help. Bracing herself with a stiff upper lip, she agreed that she could, so I assisted her to sit at the edge of the bed and dangle her feet over the side. While her blood pressure equalized, I set up the wheelchair, in true PT form, perpendicular to the gurney on the side of her good leg, removed the footrests, and locked the brakes. "I'm so dry," she rasped as she cautiously ran her tongue around her mouth. "Did something happen to my teeth? They feel jagged . . . and my throat's so sore, too."

My heart constricted with pity as I looked at her vulnerable, dear face. "They had a little trouble with the tube, but they'll get you all fixed up in a jiffy . . . now, can you stand at all on your good leg?" She slipped from the high gurney down onto her feet, wincing as her freshly scoped leg touched down, and successfully transferred over to the wheelchair without further mishap. It felt good to be able to use my modest skills as a PT to take even this small action on her behalf. A night in the hospital and my mother was able to maintain her own oxygen saturation levels, crisis averted. We counted ourselves lucky that nothing else had gone seriously wrong, but allowed the hospital to pay for the repair of her front teeth.

~ ★ ~

"Pain is just weakness leaving the body," Sam insisted as I carefully massaged his scars. His knee was a miracle of surgical success, having endured a total of seven procedures before the age of thirty-eight. Sam was a U.S. Army Ranger and had performed countless feats of extraordinary agility and bravery over his long career in the services. His left knee had originally undergone a partial meniscectomy to remove a torn, damaged meniscus on first the medial and then the lateral side of the joint during various training exercises. Then, he had managed to dislocate the patella during a parachuting accident, which ultimately required a lateral release of the iliotibial band. When he returned to work, this injury was followed by an avulsion tear of the quadriceps tendon during a covert operation, which necessitated a tendon repair, and so on. Having had his joint surfaces resculpted more than once, Sam was now in therapy for the delicate rehabilitation of a newly replaced knee joint. He was familiar with my tactics, since I had helped him recover from a previous shoulder injury in the past.

"I thought that was the slogan for the U.S. Marines," I teased as I rolled the delicate tissues beneath the pads of my fingers. I was in a tricky situation. I needed to apply enough pressure to help Sam stretch the knee, without giving him so much force that his quadriceps tendon would give way again. Beads of sweat rolled down Sam's temples as I released the tight connective tissues beneath his recent incision, but in typical noble military fashion he said nothing. "OK, Sam, let's see if we can get you to lie on your stomach for awhile so I can have my way with you," I said as I patted the treatment table under his knee. Sam grimaced but obediently turned over for me, reaching for the wad of towels I held ready for him—he sweated buckets when in pain, but never made a sound.

"Are you sure my tendon will hold up to this?" he asked as he got comfortable on his face.

"No problem," I reassured him as I grabbed hold of his ankle in preparation to bend his knee. "I've dealt with hundreds of these, and I've never broken one yet! Of course, there's always a first time for everything . . ." My confident words belied my own concern. It was a delicate task to bend his knee enough without overly stressing his previously damaged tendon.

"It feels like it wants to explode out the front," Sam said in muffled tones as I carefully mobilized his knee.

"That's what they all say," I reassured him as I continued my insistent pressure. "Now, give me a tiny outward pressure as if you're trying to straighten the knee . . . no, even smaller . . . just *think* pressure, and that'll be enough. Good, now hold five counts . . . and relax. Let me push you a little now. Great! And, repeat," I instructed as we worked carefully together on contract-relax techniques to increase the extensibility and relaxation of the contractile tissues.

Finally, I sat him up again to remeasure the knee flexion. One hundred and ten degrees—he was making great progress for such a big guy. Sam was wonderful at following up on everything I asked of him, and was the ultimate warrior who responded well to my dry wit, respect for his profession, and practical

approach. Military personnel are among my favorite types of patients, as they are
the most motivated, interesting, and heroic people I know.

When Sam finally healed and headed off to semi-retirement away from the
active military life, he presented me with a medal from the United States
Department of the Army with the slogan "Persuasive in Peace—Invincible in
War" along with a personalized plaque reading "To Anne Ahlman. Thank you
for the torture and pain—the left knee and shoulder will never be the same.
Sam." I was touched and honored, secure in the knowledge that Sam wasn't
being sarcastic. The rewards of patient care are many, but it is especially satisfying to successfully ease a person suffering from many complications back into
wellness. There is a fine line between not pushing someone hard enough and
pushing too much—this is the art of being a PT.

~ ★ ~

My husband and I have a companionable habit of going out for a casual dinner
on Saturday nights followed by a leisurely visit to the local bookstore. Once
inside the bookstore, we split apart to examine the latest offerings in new fiction,
nonfiction, music, and health and medicine. Somehow, we finish up our respective browsing at the same time and find each other among the stacks before
grabbing a decaffeinated latte and heading for home.

Tonight was no exception. We had just been to a German restaurant and
enjoyed a delicious meal of potato pancakes washed down with huge, frothy
mugs of Oktoberfest beer before our literary jaunt, and consequently I needed
to avail myself of the facilities once safely in the bookstore. Normally I avoid
using a public restroom like the plague for reasons of infection control, but this
time the good German beer had the upper hand. When I gingerly approached
the dubious-looking sink for the necessary hand washing procedure following
the recommended Centers for Disease Control and Prevention guidelines, I
stepped around another lady coming in. Without looking at her, I murmured
my apologies for being in her way and was brought up short as she exclaimed,
"I know you . . . it's Anne, right? How are you doing?" I peered at her uncomprehendingly, and then realized she was one of my old patients—I distinctly
remembered a puffy right knee, complete with hypomobile patella and tight,
reactive iliotibial band—but what was her name?

"Hi!" I stuttered, fruitlessly racking my brain. "How have you been . . . and
how is your knee doing these days?" I could definitely remember that her right

knee was riddled with arthritis, and that it had frequently swelled in response to too much walking and standing. However, she looked great and had a cute new haircut. What the heck was her name?

As we exchanged pleasantries, I remembered another vital piece of information: she owned a pet duck named Jemima, and we had often talked about Jemima's habit of flying onto the roof of the patient's house despite her clipped wings. By this time, we had maneuvered out of the restroom and were standing in the music section of the bookstore. I could see my husband patiently hovering in the background as he watched me with an amused expression. He could tell that I had no idea what this kind lady's name was, and knew I wouldn't be able to make any introductions.

Finally, I gave up. I gave my wonderful duck lady my updated clinic information, hugged her good-bye with my regards to Jemima, and rejoined my husband. "One of these days you'll just have to admit that you don't remember their names," he scolded. "It's no big deal, and it happens to everyone . . . but what I can't understand is how you remember their personal details, which body parts you helped them with, and even the names of their pets without knowing who they are!"

In retrospect, I am quite sure that if I had been able to touch the duck lady's knee, I would have remembered who she was. Many times I have been unable to remember the details of a person's injury, let alone her name, until I actually touch the affected body part again; it's as if the muscle memory in my hands remembers what my conscious brain has long since forgotten. However, it is always humbling to be greeted kindly by patients when I run across them during my travels around the city, and I am honored that they remember me.

~ ★ ~

I connected with one of my seemingly grumpy older patients over his pet. When I first met Charles, he was seated next to his gorgeous wife, who displayed a pair of high, imposing cheekbones and an elegant diamond on the ring finger of her left hand. Her rich mahogany hair was expensively styled into a sleek bob, and she was nervously chewing her lower lip. On closer inspection I could see that she had dark circles of sleeplessness and anxiety smudged beneath her eyes, and she was apprehensive about what amount of pain I might be about to inflict upon her beloved husband. Charles himself was chewing gum and humming tunelessly, protectively caged in behind a front-wheeled walker with a thick bandage wrapped

around his stiff left knee. There was an invisible, seemingly impenetrable wall bar-
ricading him from me, and I could see that the keys to his kingdom came
through Trish, his wife.

I greeted Charles pleasantly and asked how he was feeling after his recent total
knee replacement. He shot me an incredulous look as if to say how stupid was I,
couldn't I see it hurt? Misgivings aside, he allowed me to steer him across to the
treatment table, his operated leg sinking beneath him as he slowly navigated the
three-foot distance from his chair. I began the familiar routine of measuring his
initial baseline knee range of motion, and was appalled to see that his extension
was minus 25 degrees and his flexion only 78 degrees. This was one stiff knee. The
circumferential swelling was four centimeters larger than the right knee, within the
normal range of postsurgical edema. As I observed, measured, and palpated
Charles's knee, I asked him what his occupation was and if he had any particular
hobbies he wanted to return to when the knee had healed. Charles looked at me
condescendingly but admitted he was now retired and that he loved to play golf.
Again, conversation dropped to the floor like a stone. I enquired what Charles's
previous occupation was, and he responded by naming a large aerospace company.
"Oh, that sounds interesting," I said. "What did you do there?"

"I ran it," said Charles, returning to his gum and inviting no further comment.

Inwardly I sighed, recognizing that it was difficult to get along with every
patient. I strengthened my resolve to do my best for his poor knee, and began to
gently mobilize the joint. The joint was extremely stiff and felt as if it hadn't been
moved at all since the surgery three weeks ago. "Did you use a CPM on this knee
after the surgery?" I asked. The CPM, or continuous passive motion machine, is
designed to keep the knee gently moving into flexion and extension for several
hours a day to enhance circulation and reduce stiffness. Charles replied, "Yeah, I
did that for awhile, but I gave it up; the knee was so painful." We would have a
long road to travel to improve this knee, Charles and I.

Over subsequent treatments Trish came with Charles each time to watch
over him, although she visibly blanched every time I pressed Charles's knee into
its end ranges of flexion and extension. I soon learned that when Charles was
anticipating pain, he would hum. When he was feeling a painful stretch, he
would stop chewing his gum. And, when the pain became intolerable, he would
look to the sides as if scanning for arriving help, and then crack a joke. Although
we fell into a rhythm with treatment, Charles remained distant until the topic of
pets came into the conversation. At this, Charles told me all about his favorite
dog, a Labrador, who had seemed smarter than most people. As I listened eagerly

while pushing on Charles's leg, he recounted many happy trips and interactions with his pet. We agreed that one of the most unconditionally rewarding relationships in life can come through the love of a loyal pet, and from that point on we began to connect.

The knee began to respond, and Charles began to become compliant with his home exercise program for stretching under Trish's watchful eye. Then one day, the gum chewing seemed more interrupted than usual and the knee felt different under my mobilizing hands. What could it be? The swelling had come down since the initial evaluation and the color of the knee was normal, except for one small red spot blushing on the lateral aspect. The knee had become more reactive to my touch overnight, especially when I bent it as he lay prone. I joked with Charles that the knee was afraid of me now—"familiarity breeds contempt"—but asked him to describe exactly how the pain felt from his point of view. "It feels hot," he said. My stomach lurched in fear. I had noticed long ago that patients are usually extremely accurate when it comes to describing the underlying problem, and this description coupled with the feel of the knee from my perspective could mean only one thing. It was infected. There was no time to lose. I told him of my suspicions and hustled him off the table, bundling him off to the surgeon's office as quickly as possible. I scribbled a hurried progress note, faxed it to the surgeon with my suspicions, and settled down to wait with foreboding.

A day or two passed before I received a message from Trish. At first the surgeon had been unimpressed with my fears, but kindly ordered some blood work and aspirated fluid from the joint in good faith. The joint fluid looked normal, but when the lab work came back, Charles was immediately whisked off to surgery to have the joint cleaned out and was hospitalized to begin a series of extremely potent intravenous antibiotics. My fears were founded; Charles's knee was proven to be infected. This is usually not the surgeon's fault but is an incidental occurrence in the operating theater that affects a small proportion of the population. Charles was one of the unlucky ones, despite having the most thoughtful, careful, and skilled orthopedic surgeon I have ever known. But, if the spread of infection could be stopped, they would be able to save the knee. (A previous patient had described her experience with a ferocious staphylococcus aureus infection after her knee had been replaced—it turned out that the hospital nurse had accidentally cross-contaminated her wound with her roommate's, and she had narrowly avoided having the leg amputated to save her life as a result).

The powerful antibiotics destroyed Charles's bone marrow and he became so anemic and weak that Trish gently teased him by calling him "Casper." It was touch and go for weeks, but after the initial hospital treatment, Charles was sent home to continue his intravenous antibiotics and to return to physical therapy. Miraculously, I felt a huge difference in the knee's response when Charles returned, and although it wasn't exactly malleable, it was markedly less reactive. We had turned the corner. From that point on, progress was slow and steady as Charles began to experience normal amounts of pain and was able to tolerate strengthening exercises in addition to mobilization of the joint. As we soldiered on toward achieving his goals, I became curious. "How would you describe the pain you're feeling as I bend it now?" I asked as I pressed Charles's ankle toward his buttocks. The gum stilled in his mouth as he considered the question. "Just a little stiff," he said as I broke into a smile of relief.

~ ★ ~

One of my most splendidly troublesome patients came to me under circumstances similar to Charles's. Larry was instructed to see me by his orthopedic surgeon after progress with his total knee replacement rehabilitation at another physical therapy clinic had stagnated. Larry's surgeon was familiar with my tough love approach, and I had been fortunate to be able spare several of his patients further surgery through my roughshod talents with joint mobilization.

Larry was a tall man with a shock of white hair who must have been a lady-killer in his youth, but his handsome presence was spoiled by his halting gait pattern. He looked normal enough when statically sitting or standing, but when he walked it was as if the natural articulation of his left knee joint had been replaced with a stout, stiff, warped two-by-four. Larry had already undergone one manipulation under anesthesia in an attempt to unlock his stubborn knee but remained no further ahead than he had been before receiving the prosthesis. He admitted that he had no idea how important it was to move the knee around immediately after surgery, and told me that his first PT was "very sweet, but didn't push me at all." Poor Larry was in for a rough, relentless ride, because not only do I know how hard I must push on stubborn knee adhesions, but I also refuse to easily give up on people.

At first I thought that Larry was a smart, wily old bugger. Despite his permanently crooked knee, he towered over me with a long-suffering look on his face and the aroma of his favorite licorice candy on his breath. Larry projected an imposing persona, but I couldn't see beyond his poor leg, which looked like he had stolen it from a stork—the quadriceps and calf muscles were atrophied and flat, yet the knee joint itself was rudely swollen and thick. When I measured his initial knee range of motion, I found that he was stuck close to 30 degrees, the loose-pack position of the joint. In this position the joint surfaces are at their most open orientation, which allows for the greatest comfort, especially when swelling is an issue; unfortunately, Larry's knee appeared to have become glued there. "They told me I should've had this surgery over ten years ago," Larry commented as I made faces over the state of his leg. "In fact, when I consulted with an orthopedic team back home in Indiana, the surgeons asked me where my wheelchair was, because after they saw the X-rays they thought it would be impossible for such a wrecked knee to be walked on!"

"So what took you so long?" I asked. "Hasn't it been increasingly hard to get around?"

"Well, it wasn't so bad until my golf game started to suffer," he said with a grin. "I was doing fine with using the cart and everything, but I found out that I couldn't pivot anymore through that leg and I was getting nowhere near the green . . . so, I thought I'd better finally go through with it. My surgeon's great, but I guess things were pretty complicated once he got in there, because he found a big cyst in the bone behind my knee. He tried to cut it out, but he warned me that the recovery might be pretty tough." Here he paused to grimace as I attempted to bend the leg. "Man that hurts! I don't think these narcotics are even touching it . . . and it seems no better than before the manipulation."

"Have you been stretching the knee on a daily basis?" I asked.

"Nah, not really—it's just been too sore to move. The only thing that feels really good is the ice," he replied.

My heart sank. All that suffering and no progress! In my experience, stiff post-surgical joints do best with frequent input. Because knees are fairly stoic in their response to stretching, I always advise my patients to nag their knees to death on an hourly basis, working the knee into flexion on the hour and then pushing it into extension on the half hour. If knees don't get repeated stretching, they can freeze in a hurry. It's similar to attempting to keep cement from setting—you have to keep stirring it, or it will harden fast. Of course, patients aren't able to push the limb as strongly as I can since I have the advantage of leverage, but they can really help themselves maintain the gains we make together during our therapy visits by keeping things moving.

Larry was back at square one. I delivered my customary lecture about the importance of constantly moving the joint into end ranges, and began mobilizing the knee. I set up stabilizing towels to use as a fulcrum beneath Larry's leg, took up the slack of his soft tissues, and pressed the knee into extension until my fingers blanched—nothing happened. I applied more pressure, upgrading the force of my mobilization from a grade II to a grade IV (end range pressure). The entire dorsal surface of my hands turned white. Hmm. I rearranged the towels, checked Larry's status (everything felt excruciating to him, despite the heavy duty narcotics onboard), and tried again. After several minutes of careful, sweaty oscillation, my hands fell asleep, so I called a halt and measured his extension. It had improved from minus 30 degrees to minus 24 degrees, so we were painfully on the right track.

Larry and I took a sweat-mopping break, and then I had him turn onto his stomach. "I haven't tried to lie on my stomach since before the surgery," he protested weakly.

"Well, let's just try it—if it's too painful, we'll try something else. But, if you can tolerate the position, it can be very successful," I encouraged. Over the years innumerable patients have come to me after failing to improve their stiff knees at other therapy clinics, and I have found that many of them never had their knees bent in a way that allowed proper stretching of the quadriceps muscle and its attachments. Too many therapists would work on knee flexion in a seated position when the quadriceps is slack, and thus the anterior muscles and associated surgical adhesions would remain rigid. If patients can comfortably be positioned prone or even lying on their sides with a straight hip and thigh alignment, the therapist can then employ a different approach to help stretch the soft tissues around the knee.

I padded Larry's knee by placing a towel roll beneath his thigh, so that the patella would not grind into the treatment bench, and began to stretch him. At a mere 45 degrees of flexion, licorice-laced moans began to escape from Larry's compressed lips as he heroically clenched his teeth. His knee was unbelievably stiff, but since I could feel some give in the tissues, I carefully persisted. After I felt that we could both take no more, I asked Larry to sit up so that I could remeasure his knee flexion. The knee was now able to bend up to 80 degrees, which was markedly better than his initial flexion measurement of barely 65 degrees.

And so it went. Larry showed up in good faith three days a week to endure my little torture routine. "The doctor says that if anyone can get this knee to come around, it'll be you," he would say cheerfully before submitting to my tender mercies. Each session was an exercise in pain for us both—Larry said he was only aware of a red haze of agony as I massaged, mobilized, bent, and otherwise mangled his knee, and I felt as if my hands and even my shoulders were about to part from my body in a burning firefall as I struggled to find an unbruised portion of myself with which to push against him. Since I was only too painfully aware of the discomfort I routinely inflicted upon him, I always treated Larry in a treatment room instead of the more public gym area to help keep his agonized yodeling private.

One day as Larry and I staggered out of the treatment room together, rearranging our respective clothing, the receptionist sidled up to us, giggling. "Didn't you hear me out in the hall earlier?" she asked with a hint of mischief sparkling in her eyes. "I don't know exactly what you were doing in there, but I was showing a prospective client and her husband around the facility when Larry let out a terrible roar of pain—the clients looked at each other with horrified expressions and fled! I doubt we'll ever see them again."

As the weeks passed, it became only too apparent that Larry's knee could stretch just so far—he would have to have a second manipulation if he were to ever comfortably walk the golf course again. At that time I was working in clinical patient care only in the mornings, as I devoted my afternoons to my medical writing work, but I gave Larry my cell phone number so that he could contact me. Finally, the day of his second manipulation dawned, and we coordinated our schedules: Larry would phone me as soon as he woke up from anesthesia, and I would meet him in the clinic to resume working on his leg. This time, we were able to move his knee quickly and aggressively, and over the ensuing weeks, Larry tolerated my ministrations five times a week to take advantage of his freshly manipulated joint. Finally, we were able to taper our frequency of treatment and the potency of Larry's pain medication (although we had been concerned about a possible addiction to the narcotics, Larry was made of sterner stuff), and he was walking like a new man.

The first time Larry achieved 120 degrees of knee flexion, he celebrated by bringing a bottle of champagne in for me. (How did he know?) Once he returned to the golf course, he realized that he was playing better than ever, since he was able to weight bear and pivot through the offending knee properly. "I can drive the ball further than I could before the surgery!" he exclaimed in excited tones. Other golfers who had also been patients of mine reported that Larry had a "sweet" stroke, and could hit a long ball. The only problem was that the right knee, which also needed to be replaced, was causing him to limp and was holding him back from easily clambering out of the sand traps.

Larry decided to hold off for as long as possible in order to enjoy his newfound therapy-free existence, but cagily asked what my retirement plans were.

I mischievously reassured him, "For your sake, I hope I don't see you again in the clinic for a good, long time—but just in case, we won't have our house paid off for another ten years." Fortunately, Larry's right knee replacement just two years later went according to plan.

A Well-Turned Ankle

May those that love us, love us;
And those that don't love us, may God turn their hearts.
And if He doesn't turn their hearts, may He turn their ankles
so we will know them by their limping.
—*Irish Blessing*

We think of our ankles as simple hinge joints, but they actually consist of two distinct bony articulations. The upper "true" ankle joint that allows up and down movements of the foot comprises the ends of the two lower leg bones, the tibia and fibula, which glide against the ankle's talus bone beneath them. The talus provides the connection between the lower leg and the foot. The two protruding bones that we normally associate with the ankle are really the ends of the tibia (medial malleolus) and the fibula (lateral malleolus). It is between these two bones that the talus rests. The true ankle joint is at its most stable when the foot is flat on the floor or mildly dorsiflexed, because in this position the talus is physically closer to the stabilizing bones of the tibia and fibula as the ankle moves. The ankle joint is least stable when the foot is plantar flexed, because in this position there is more space between the three bones of the true ankle joint; here, the ankle is much more vulnerable to unanticipated movement and must rely primarily on the surrounding ligaments and tendons to hold it together. This is why it is so much easier to sprain your ankle when you're pointing your toes, such as occurs when taking a misstep when running or when wearing high heels.

The subtalar joint is the second ankle articulation that is the junction of the talus and the calcaneus, or heel bone, beneath. This lower joint is the area where sideways movements of the ankle occur. The two joints of the ankle complex are held in check by a system of restraining ligaments on the inside and outside of the ankle. We call stretching or breaking a ligament an ankle sprain, which is the most common injury of the ankle region. With sprains, the most frequently injured ligament is the anterior talofibular ligament, which is the ligament that spans the distance between the talus and the front part of the fibula at the lateral ankle. Other support ligaments that may be damaged with a severe inversion sprain are also located at the lateral ankle, including the calcaneofibular and posterior talofibular ligaments.

Occasionally, the medial ankle may also become sprained (eversion sprain) despite the relative strength of the large triangular deltoid ligament that holds the medial malleolus to the talus. Any sprain that occurs with enough force can also rupture the syndesmotic ligament, a tough membrane that connects the tibia to the fibula. Because of their relatively poor blood supply, ligaments heal quite slowly and are prone to re-injury once damaged. Usually, once a ligament has been sprained it becomes permanently stretched from its original shape, allowing the ankle even more motion and potential for further damage.

Since most of us walk, jog, dance, and run more than a million steps each year, it is likely that at some time in our lives we will experience ankle stress and pain. We sometimes call spraining an ankle "turning an ankle," which is different from displaying a shapely ankle, also known as a well-turned ankle. Historically, ankles have been thought to represent femininity and were once considered a scandalous sight if they were caught peeking out from beneath a woman's petticoats.

~ ★ ~

Tamara was set to stumble along in her ancestors' footsteps just like the rest of us. When I first met her, Tamara was an awkward, uncoordinated thirteen-year-old who had been pushed into competitive soccer and swimming by an over-ambitious mother. Her mother was bored, fancied herself as Tamara's friend and confidante, and strove to dress and act like a teenager herself. "Isn't it funny that Tamara and I can share the same clothes?" she would giggle annoyingly as she performed hyperactive push-ups on the treatment room floor while I attempted to concentrate on treating Tamara's ankle. Tamara simply rolled her eyes and returned to text messaging her friends on her cell phone, oblivious to her mother's antics.

Tamara had severely sprained her ankle, involving not only the anterior talofibular ligament, but also the posterior talofibular and deltoid ligaments. The peroneal tendons just behind the lateral malleolus were also strained. But how had she done so much damage? Tamara had been going through a growth spurt and was heavily encouraged to play soccer and attend swim practice every day despite feelings of fatigue or pain. Eventually, when Tamara encountered an uneven soccer pitch, the tired dynamic stabilizer muscles in her lower leg were unable to adequately control her ankle movement and she fell, spraining the supportive straplike ligaments around the ankle. Tamara initially reported sharp eight out of ten pain at both the medial and lateral aspects of the ankle, and could walk only when using a brace and crutches. When it comes to ankle sprains, the research on the difference between boys and girls indicates that boys sprain their ankles primarily due to tight, restricted soft tissues around the ankle, but that with growth spurts, girls have a slowed proprioceptive response that leaves their ankles more vulnerable to injury.

It didn't help that Tamara, in her gangly, growing way, had poor body awareness and could not (or would not) follow directions. She was impossible to treat, as she could not distinguish between a feeling of fatigue and actual pain, a concept we revisited time and time again. During the first month of therapy, Tamara began to improve but said she was frustrated by her relative inactivity and was unable to stop herself from exercising through her pain. After I advised Tamara to stay out of the pool, off her bicycle, and on her brace and crutches to allow healing to take place, Tamara came back in to say that her mother had hauled her off to an osteopathic doctor for an adjustment because she was sure Tamara's ankle was "out."

"Out where?" I asked in genuine confusion.

"Out of position. The doctor said that my ankle was dislocated, and that he put it back," she responded.

"It couldn't be dislocated, or you wouldn't be able to walk on it! Besides, your orthopedic surgeon has done a bunch of X-rays and everything looked normal—no dislocation, fracture, or bone chip—so if the ankle were 'out' it would have shown up," I said. "So, now is it 'in'? If so, does it feel all better?"

"It just feels weird," Tamara said. "Kinda sore and wobbly."

Her long-suffering orthopedic surgeon decided to put Tamara into a walking boot to try to stabilize the persistently painful ankle. In response, Tamara decided to take the boot off at a school dance and jig around with her friends for three hours, slamming down onto her injured stockinged foot while she wore a high heel on the other foot. Predictably, she got worse. Her resolute orthopedist then put her in a walking cast for one month to ensure that the soft tissues could finally rest and heal without continued re-injury, reasoning that the hard cast would be impossible to take off. At last, things improved.

Tamara wasn't a bad kid, just a confused one who was continually trying to please her mother, her coaches, and her peers, against medical orders and her own best interests. During therapy, Tamara would put down her cell phone and talk about all sorts of things from the pressures of sports and schoolwork to her self-imposed role as psychologist to her friends and family.

As I slowly helped Tamara normalize her ankle responses with proprioceptive neuromuscular facilitation (PNF) patterns, balance activities, and careful strengthening after the cast came off, I reflected that the PT's role often includes that of counselor and mentor, especially with children who find it difficult to relate to their parents during the adolescent years.

~ ★ ~

Sadly, my ankles have never been considered well turned. They are as thick and sturdy and durable as I am, so much so that in the face of injury they have chosen to become increasingly stiff and stubborn, rather than becoming looser and more pliable. It seems that spraining an ankle is a rite of passage for most humans, and I am no exception. The first time it happened to me was well after I had graduated from college.

I was riding my valiant Irish thoroughbred Riley in a jumping competition on the polo fields at Golden Gate Park in San Francisco. Our first class went like a dream, Riley winning the Governor's Cup after accurately cutting corners in the jump-off against the clock. It was one of those rounds when two hearts beat as one, and we flew around the course, leaving out strides and jumping the fences at impossible angles to beat the competition. Later that day, we were sedately cantering between the fourth and fifth fences of our second event when Riley slipped on the fog-dampened grass and fell, pinning my right ankle beneath his sturdy ribs. Although I cushioned him from the worst of the impact, poor Riley ended up with a large hematoma on his hip, and I sustained a severely sprained ankle, which would have been much worse without the support of my stiff leather riding boot.

Eventually, the scar tissue I laid down when healing from the accident served to permanently restrict my ability to dorsiflex my right foot at the ankle. This has been a nuisance when trying to fully get my heels down in the stirrups when riding, and forces me to ride with my right stirrup a half-hole longer than the left. However, at this point my right ankle became immune to further sprains, freeing my left ankle up for misbehavior. Although it had enjoyed an injury-free childhood, the left ankle finally collapsed beneath me with a shriek when it collided with one of my husband's shoes as it lay parked at the foot of the stairs . . . now I have a matched set of ankles.

~ ★ ~

The fingernails on Frank's right hand were overly long and filthy, immediately catching my eye and throwing me into a flurry of indecision. Did I have to shake his hand when I greeted him? Could I just smile and quickly turn my attention to his leg instead?

Frank was a weekend warrior who had been playing softball with friends when someone unexpectedly hit him in the calf with one of the bats, making Frank fall to the ground. As he lay there groaning in pain, Frank found that there had been no one near him after all—his Achilles tendon had partially torn all on its own, and it had just felt as if someone had assaulted him. Frank was more fortunate than most, since the tendon fibers had torn at the musculo-tendinous junction instead of at the tendon itself, and he was still able to walk, albeit with crutches.

Frank's lower calf was an impressively gory blend of bright and dark-red bruises interspersed with tones of deepening purple. It was immensely swollen, but his MRI report had shown only a 25 percent thickness tear of the medial gastrocnemius muscle at the proximal part of the Achilles tendon, with the majority of the tendon fortunately unharmed. Frank was one of the lucky ones and would not need to have surgery. However, due to his apprehension, Frank was completely unable to even place his toes on the floor in case the tendon might choose to fully rupture, and was hobbling around on his heel, without engaging his calf muscle, in a sweat of fear. His surgeon had sent him over to therapy to try to help Frank relearn how to walk despite his anxiety.

It transpired that Frank played guitar in his spare time when away from the law office and softball field, thus the super-long fingernails on his right hand. I teased him gently that he could at least keep his nails clean if they had to be long, but the joke was lost on him. "Long fingernails are the badge of an artist," he insisted. "I need these nails to pluck the guitar strings, and it's not the same sound if I use a guitar pick." Ugh.

After measuring Frank's ankle range of motion (full passive range but minus 20 degrees of dorsiflexion and only 30 degrees of plantar flexion when measured actively), I asked him to roll onto his stomach on the treatment bench so I could clearly examine the injured ankle and calf. He was extremely reluctant to do so, and began to sweat profusely. "I have an extremely high threshold for pain," Frank explained, "but you have no idea how much this hurts . . . in fact, I don't think you should be touching it directly until it gets better; just show me the exercises I need to do." I explained that it would be important for me to gently feel the injured region in order to determine where the areas of worst damage were to help me focus my treatment with ultrasound and soft tissue mobilization. With musculotendinous injuries, the name of the game is to enhance circulation to the area, since blood flow brings oxygen to the tissues, and oxygenation speeds the healing process. In addition, since injured muscles and tendons will often attempt to heal in a shortened position, it is imperative to carefully stretch the soft tissues throughout the recovery process or risk facing re-injury when returning to normal life.

Frank wanted none of it, and it was only after sympathetic yet firm cajoling that I could get him to lie down at all. When I first approached his calf, I used a touch similar to that of a small sickly child petting a hummingbird. Regardless, Frank leapt off the table in consternation. "That's a seven out of ten pain right there," he cried. I silently handed him a towel to sop up his nervous sweat. I knew that the regions of the lower calf and ankle that showed the greatest amount of bruising were unlikely to harbor the worst damage, since gravity pulls blood toward the ground with time; therefore, as I carefully palpated Frank's injured lower leg and ankle, I focused on the areas directly above the scenic sunset. Here, I could feel several areas of increased tissue density that I knew would be exquisitely painful but decided to save these areas to apply the ultrasound to first, knowing that this would remove the worst sting from being touched. Despite all my care, Frank continued to cower like a naughty puppy at the very lightest of my examining touches.

As I used ultrasound and then gently began to work on Frank's calf and ankle, he finally relaxed a little bit into my pressure and began to cross-examine me about my experience as a PT and about his own reactions to therapy. "How can you tell where the injury is?" he asked. "I suppose the big bruises are one indication, but I don't have a lot of pain where those are. It seems impossible that you could sense the most painful areas, and yet every time you came to an especially sore spot you asked me if the area hurt before I could even react. How do you do it?"

I explained to him that PTs develop palpation skills over years of experience with various injuries, and quoted a few bits of research to him to gain his trust. Frank's demeanor toward me started to soften and become less defensive as I established credibility in his mind. As we talked, he became quite eager to know how he stacked up against all the other patients I had seen over the years. "I've always known that I have a high tolerance for pain," he began, "But I really want to know if you agree with that, having seen so many patients and being able to compare my performance against theirs. How does my pain tolerance measure up with other guys?"

My probing fingers stopped for a moment as I considered Frank's question. What on earth could I say that was truthful but wouldn't hurt his feelings? In my opinion, his pain tolerance was relatively poor: he was very reactive, he cried out at even the lightest touch, and he complained about how much it hurt despite my detailed explanations of what we were doing and why. However, he did let me continue treatment despite his pain and anxiety.

I simply couldn't lie to him, so I cautiously started, "Frank, we're here now together doing whatever we can to speed the healing process. Why does it matter how other people react? Everyone's different and has had different experiences that contribute to their reactions. Besides, everyone knows women are much tougher than men!" I joked. But Frank wouldn't let it go, and twisted his upper body around so that he could see my expression from his prone position. "Yes, yes—I'm sure," he said. "But, really, I want to know how I measure up . . . and for the sake of comparison, take all those tough women out of the equation," he insisted, his flinty gaze never leaving my face.

"Frank, your pain tolerance is better than some, and not as good as others," I replied. "What matters is that you're a smart guy who is able to override his fear of pain with logic—even though you feel that my touch is painful to you, you understand that it will help you heal as quickly as possible. You know, of course, that the definition of courage is to face your fears even though you feel that you are about to confront something that is difficult or painful. I think that in the end, being brave is much more valuable than having a high pain tolerance, because it takes a strong quality of spirit, whereas a high pain tolerance is a passive thing."

Frank said no more, but lapsed into a reflective silence. From that moment on, he let me do anything I liked to help his treatment along and no longer complained of pain. The idea of being courageous in the face of pain actually increased his pain threshold to a level he could be proud of.

Forces of Nature

Heaven is under our feet, as well as over our heads.

—Henry David Thoreau, American author, naturalist, and philosopher
(1817–1862)

The feet are our most fundamental link to the earth that we stand on, and serve to ground us in our daily lives. This connection means different things to many people, and the feet may be despised or appreciated depending on their appearance (although only a podiatrist truly can be grateful for certain characteristics of the aging foot). Feet can be a pedestrian means of getting from A to B, springs with which to run and kick and hike, forms upon which to display pretty footwear, or smelly dogs with gnarled, yellow toenails to be hidden from the world's view. Those of us with merely ordinary feet are hard-pressed to find many details with which to wax poetic until we meet people without the luxury of such mundane, functional items.

In addition to performing the most obvious of functions, the feet are actually sensitive antennae that give us unlimited amounts of information about where we stand, and are essential components of the somatosensory system. Some of us are ticklish and some are not; somehow, like the half-and-half distribution of my palmaris longus, my left foot is ticklish, but my right foot is as serene as an unruffled lake to the touch of another.

~ ★ ~

My husband teases me that I have duck feet. I sport the same high arches, wide ball of the foot, elongated second toes, and slightly turned-in aspect that my English grandmother had. Already burdened with a triple-E shoe width by the age of eight, I was taken to a podiatrist by my mother, who was desperate to remedy the unsightly problem. After all, I could fit only into sandals (which I had to wear with socks to keep my circulation active in chilly San Francisco), since ordinary shoes pinched terribly. The good doctor looked me over, commented that I was born to walk on a beach, and suggested that if I didn't concentrate on walking with my feet pointing straight ahead instead of looking at each other, he would break them and reset them for me. I have yet to discover how much this brief consultation cost my parents, but it was effective—though they are even wider now, my feet point resolutely forward as I walk. I have since discovered that the shape of my feet hark back to a robust Viking origin, and feel pleased that my high, supinated arches prevent pain during the long hours of standing at work.

~ ★ ~

"You really enjoy hurting people, don't you?" sneered Mandy as I pushed deeply into the plantar fascia on the bottom of her right foot. My thumbs were on fire, my forearms were burning unpleasantly with lactic acid, and my fingers had become bright red throbbing sausages in my efforts to help her mobilize and stretch the contracted fascial connective tissue. White hot rage flared up in my heart as I recoiled from her unjust accusation. I knew that one of the best ways to stretch tight, painful plantar fascial tissue was to apply ultrasound to improve the extensibility of the deep tissues and then perform manual deep tissue mobilization to help elongate the fibers. I was hurting myself in my supreme efforts to help this ungrateful woman, but I stuffed my anger back down.

I sat back on my stool and looked Mandy squarely in the eye. "Actually, I'd much rather be sitting in my garden reading an interesting novel with a glass of wine in one hand and a box of chocolates in the other, if you really want to know. We talked about your condition and what types of treatment would be the most helpful; but, you know, this is totally up to you! If you don't want me to help you, just say so."

Mandy shrugged and looked away, the sneer still playing along her upper lip. "OK then, just a tiny bit more," I said. "Once we get this a little more malleable we can have you work on the stretches at home using a can of soda underneath your foot. It's like rolling out a piece of bread dough—you just move the arch of your foot across the can under pressure until the pain begins to recede."

No reaction. I sighed inwardly, knowing that the odds of any follow-through were slim with this patient. Plantar fasciitis was certainly an extremely unpleasant affliction, but it usually responded to physical therapy treatment, home stretching, and sometimes a splint boot to keep the bottom of the foot elongated during the night. Mandy would probably end up needing a cortisone injection in her foot. I felt sorry for the doctor who'd have to deliver it, as she'd probably kick him in the head for his trouble.

I finished my treatment session, leaving Mandy to ruminate on my apparent cruelty—the physical terrorist strikes again. Back up at the front desk, I found that my next patient was a new one. "Plantar Fasciitis" read the accompanying prescription. I groaned—two in a row! What were the odds? I cast an apologetic look at my still swollen and throbbing thumb MCP joints and strode off to meet the next patient.

~ ★ ~

Gina was an unkempt forty-something with wild, wiry hair and a general air of disorganization. Her white pants were smudged with what looked like raspberry jam, her shirt was partially untucked, and her feet were poking out from an ancient pair of Birkenstocks. The formerly tidy treatment room was littered with partially used paper cups, sections of newspaper, a grubby powder-blue sweater, and a battered brown faux leather handbag. As I knocked and entered, Gina looked up and kicked her feet down to the floor from their resting place on the treatment table as she laid down the Lifestyle section of the paper. "Hi there," she greeted me pleasantly, "I'm Gina—forgive the mess, but I'm so used to disorder I seem to create it now wherever I go! At home I'm surrounded by two little boys, and you know what they're like . . . plus, it doesn't help that they both have ADHD. It's funny, since they're not related—we adopted, you know—but they just can't seem to ever sit still or concentrate on anything!"

As Gina paused for breath, I intervened and introduced myself. As we talked on about her history of left foot pain (excruciating, worse first thing in the morning, terrible after sitting too long, etc.), I glanced down at the offending foot. Despite being tucked into its lair within the nasty old scuffed Birkenstock sandal, I could see that it was absolutely filthy. After explaining that I would need to manually assess her foot, I invited Gina to come and wash her foot in our sink before beginning. "No, I'm fine," she said as she kicked off her sandal and shoved her dirty foot under my nose. "I think it would be best," I said. "We'll probably use ultrasound on the foot, and it might push any particles of dirt from your skin into the deeper tissues, so it's really best to start with a clean foot."

"No, really, I finally got comfortable here. I haven't sat down in days, and I don't want to get up again, so I'll take my chances," she laughed.

What to do? Should I risk offending her by putting on gloves or by scrubbing her foot with a damp, hot towel? What if she complained to the clinic owner about my apparent rudeness? But must I be subjected to touching and inhaling the rank scent of her dirty foot while I worked on it?

In the interest of time, I held my breath and plunged into treatment. Usually, my worst foot patients are unwashed teenage boys who attend PT straight after football practice without the benefit of a shower. On Gina, the ultrasound gel mixed with cortisone cream that was usually a delicate shade of light blue predictably turned dark gray as I moved the sound head across the underside of her foot. My stomach heaved—the smell was like a thousand dirty socks that had been dragged through a fraternity house bathroom after an all-night party. Nonetheless, I completed the phonophoresis treatment and wiped her foot thoroughly before attempting to touch the foot with my own hands. The towel came away a peculiar shade of brown, reminiscent of the contents of bags of steer manure at the garden center.

On Gina's following visit, the same whirlwind greeted me when I opened the door. Her keys were dangling from the edge of the counter where she had flung them, and as I walked inside, something crunched unpleasantly under my feet. There, crumbling on the previously pristine, gleaming linoleum floor were innumerable dirt clods and other grimy bits of debris. Gina's Birkenstocks were freshly bathed in a layer of caked, drying mud, which was the source of the mess.

"My foot felt much better after last time," she enthused.

"I'm so glad," I responded. "But—is it raining outside? You seem to have tracked some mud in with you."

"Rain, in California? In July? Silly! No, I was just watering my plants before I came over; the poor things looked like they were fading away in this heat," she said.

"Ah, I see. Well, let's get started. We really must wash your foot first now that it's all muddy," I said.

"No, no need—I'm fine—just building up my immunity, you know!" Gina cackled.

"No, really, I insist," I said. No way was I touching the offending foot in this state. "Come on, follow me; the sink is just down the hallway here, and I have a nice fresh towel all ready for you. Here, I'll even warm up the water for you!"

Gina reluctantly followed me out of the room, crunching dispiritedly in my wake. Victory! Gina's foot was a pleasing pink color beneath the encrusted filth, and I was able to treat her without fear that I was packing some horrible soil-based organisms into the tight spaces beneath my already short, tidy fingernails, or worse, driving them into her foot with the ultrasonic waves. In retrospect, I had waited too long to insist on adequate patient hygiene—although concern for myself is not the strongest motivating factor, potential harm to the patient is. Since this incident, I have taken a stronger leadership role to ensure the safety of my patients, and insist on setting up the parameters of treatment properly, regardless of a patient's temporary displeasure.

~ ★ ~

Although I am a reasonably fastidious person, I too can succumb to the forces of nature. Because of my increased-weight-bearing-on-the-left-lower-extremity habit, over time my left foot has grown longer than the right one as it has deformed in response to the daily stresses of holding me up. This length difference, combined with the natural tendency for both feet to be duckishly wide, means that I have a great deal of trouble finding shoes that fit comfortably. Over time, the great toenail of my left foot has sought refuge from uneven shoe pressure and relentless weight bearing and has retreated unappealingly toward my nail bed. This condition, otherwise known as an ingrown toenail, can be surprisingly painful.

When I finally figured out what was happening beneath my signature purple toenail polish, I decided to research the condition and treat myself. First, I painstakingly cleaned my instruments and sterilized them with rubbing alcohol to remove any undesirable bacterial hitchhikers. Then, I followed the step-by-step directions on a well-known medically peer-reviewed Web site to trim the offending nail back away from the inflamed nail bed. All went well and the pressure was alleviated, although my swollen, reddened toe skin was still sore. I painfully sluiced out the nail bed with hydrogen peroxide to clean the area, gave myself a dose of an over-the-counter anti-inflammatory medicine, and settled down to wait for my pain-free walking days to return.

Days passed and I thought that the worst was over. Weeks passed and the problem returned. Months went by and I found myself trapped in a new routine just to make it through each day—sterilize, trim, bathe in hydrogen peroxide, and chase with an antibiotic ointment to scare away the critters. The pain came and went, with some days better than others. Walking remained consistently painful, and any pressure applied to the tip of my big toe was agonizing, feeling as if hot needles were being stuck into the end of my toe. During my waking moments I remained vigilant so that no untoward pressure touched my foot, but I woke myself with a scream caught in my throat quite a few times before I learned to sleep with my left foot hanging out of the bed, away from the touch of even a light sheet. Putting on my socks was a battle of wills, but if I gave myself some extra dead space of baggy sock at the end of my toe, I could just tolerate easing my foot into my wide shoes each morning.

Six months in, I began to seriously wonder why my pain tolerance was so poor; my toe was still extremely painful, especially to direct palpation at the tip of the toe. During this time I hiked for miles, stumbled over uneven terrain to walk cross-country courses at three-day event competitions, and managed a trip to visit family in the North of England and Scotland. I stopped mentioning my pain unless I inadvertently yelped when I caught the toe against something, because complaining simply didn't change the situation.

Within a week after my husband and I arrived home from our trip to the United Kingdom, I fell ill with an unproductive cough and unrelenting fevers. After the twelfth day, I weakly joked to my husband that my toe was infected and was poisoning my whole body . . . and with a growing sense of apprehension and horror decided that I had better see a physician.

Having no personal doctor, since I was normally healthy, I staggered off to the urgent care clinic and wrote on the intake form "possible pneumonia; toe infection." After my two-hour wait, I was shown in to see a nurse practitioner who thought that I had the flu and told me to go home to bed. I doubtfully agreed, but asked that she peek at my toe while I was there, which had been becoming steadily misshapen at the tip. She looked at it, said it looked like nothing, and prepared to leave until I described my symptoms in a little more detail. After excusing herself, she returned with one of the doctors who took one look at my toe and said, "This is hugely abscessed! How did you get here without using crutches?"

He shined a light directly upon the tip of my toe, and even I could see that the toe was meanly undercut with a tight, billowing white substance. I began to flinch, feeling slightly nauseous. "Go ahead and lance it," the doctor instructed, "and then be sure to squeeze out all of the pus—it looks like the infection goes deep beneath the entire nail bed and is probably beginning to destroy the bone." With that pronouncement, he left the room with a flick of his white coat.

The nurse practitioner and I looked at each other. "This will hurt a bit," she said doubtfully.

"I know, but let's do it—maybe I'll be able to sleep with both feet inside the sheets after this!" I joked.

"You shouldn't have waited so long to come in," she chastised.

I let her comment fall to the floor, where it deserved to lie. This episode was reminiscent of the time ten years previously when I had contracted a severe bacterial pneumonia from a patient during my time working in a nursing home—back then, I was so sick that I lost ten pounds during the first seven days of constant fever, coughing, and painfully crackling lungs. Similarly, I had sought help at an urgent care center (a different one) where an overly enthusiastic nurse practitioner who had formerly been a respiratory therapist diagnosed me with allergic bronchitis. Of course, being the respiratory specialist, she was extremely self-assured about the accuracy of her diagnosis, and packed me off home armed with inhalers. I worsened by the hour and crawled back to the urgent care center the next day, insisting on seeing a doctor. I was shown into a cubicle, where I lay down sweating, short of breath, and too weak to sit. When the same nurse practitioner bustled into my cubicle I feebly raised my hand, pointed at her with a trembling index finger, and croaked, "Get out of here! I want to see a doctor!" until she left with crimson cheeks flaming. Within minutes I had an actual physician listening to my chest, taking an X-ray, and giving me the antibiotics that saved my life.

"Are you ready?" the nurse asked, her scalpel poised over my left foot. "If we must," I replied as I resolutely focused my gaze on the eye chart adhered to the opposite wall. Was that an E or an F on the fourth line? Without further ado, the nurse practitioner plunged the scalpel deeply into my distended toe with gusto as I winced acutely. A red haze of pain exploded in my head and my right foot twitched in its eagerness to get me out of there. Amazingly, I managed to keep my left foot still, if only to avoid the scalpel penetrating deeper.

"Wow—there's a TON of pus in here!" the nurse said excitedly as the stuff came pouring out all over her gloved fingers.

"Mmmph," I answered, writhing around on the treatment table while steadfastly keeping my left foot still.

"OK, I'm going to press on the toe a little—this may hurt," the nurse benignly informed me as she squeezed my toe robustly to empty out the alien fluid.

Agony. But, when the ordeal was completed my big toe was a normal size again for the first time in months. I shakily asked for after-care instructions, and received a lecture on toe hygiene. "The field of medicine has changed in its recommendations and now suggests that you no longer use hydrogen peroxide. With an abscess, just soak the toe in warm water four times a day, and then dab a little antibiotic ointment on it when it bursts. Of course, I burst this one for you, so just keep up the warm soaks and ointment until it heals so that it doesn't seal off again."

I needed no further invitation and sped off home for my first soaking session. The toe took more than three weeks to fully heal, but That Pain was gone. Unfortunately, this had no effect on my worsening respiratory illness. Back to the doctor I went (this time to a proper general internal medicine person) for chest X-rays, as the realization slowly dawned on me that unrelenting fevers plus implacable coughing must equal pneumonia. Sure enough, the blood work and X-rays revealed that I had a case of walking pneumonia—this time of viral origin—that would be unable to respond to antibiotics. Now I would be forced to rest and take better care of myself. Cursing the airlines' inadequate air recirculation system, the probable source of my illness, I endured another six weeks of the pneumonia as it slowly resolved. As an active person who is used to pushing herself relentlessly through her responsibilities and obligations, sick or well, I discovered that slowing down was the hardest part of the cure.

As I gradually regained my interest in life and my former energy levels, I found that my toe was perfect. It was a profound joy to be able to shift my weight back onto my left leg again, stabilizing myself comfortably in the familiar position that lets me use my dominant right arm freely. At last! If only I had sought help more quickly, I could have spared myself a lot of trouble. However, therapists and other health professionals are often the last people to get into the patient schedule book for treatment or even to admit that they have a problem. As a group, we are so habituated to helping others, to stepping outside of ourselves regardless of our own mental or physical wellness, and to focusing on the other person's recovery that we frequently don't take the time that we should to keep our own bodies fresh and strong.

Soon after the Great Toe/Pneumonia Debacle I vowed that from now on, things would be different. Although I would always be ready to roll up my sleeves to help another person, exposing my naked elbows as a symbol of my willingness to connect with them, I was finally ready to value myself as an integral part of that process. Although never pleasant, each injury or illness that I experience grants me more insight into my patients' feelings. Every personal interaction that I become engaged in gives me fresh appreciation for the infinite depths and innumerable facets of the human condition, and gives me fresh perspective on healing and patient care. And always, the connection of one soul with another bestows wisdom upon me and gives my life meaning.

Part Five

Reflections

The art of medicine consists of amusing the patient while Nature cures the disease.
—*François-Marie Arouet de Voltaire, French Enlightenment philosopher*
(1694–1778)

Sometimes, the most challenging patients arrive in the clinic only after becoming therapist-shy from a previous experience under a colleague's hands. But different therapists are just that—different. Despite attending accredited schools throughout the nation, therapists are individuals who arrive at the bedside with unique sets of past experiences and bags of tricks with which to help each patient through the recovery process. As therapists gain wisdom through interactions with their professors in school, instructors on clinical rotations, mentors in the workplace, fellow health professionals at continuing education courses, and the patients themselves on a daily basis, they develop an extensive array of tools and techniques that "work" for them. However, therapists are only human and can get stuck in a rut, attempting to treat a changing condition with the same techniques that worked before to no avail.

After studying a medical illustration chart depicting the musculoskeletal system, a patient recently commented that although he was quite sure it was all routine to me, he felt "in awe" of the human body. This observation gave me pause for a moment, but as I said to him that day, I realized that despite the essential sameness of our physical structures, no two people are exactly alike. Each person is a unique amalgamation of bone, muscle, tendon, ligament, fascia, nerve, and spirit that responds to similar injuries quite differently. The basic anatomy is merely a stepping-stone to discovering which singular factors of work, play, and relaxation affect the person's condition. With this in mind, I can never treat any two people the same way even if they share an identical diagnosis—nor would I want to.

The challenge and the joy of being a physical therapist is to discover how to restore each patient to his or her own special place in the world. The ability to play even a small part in the healing of another person while experiencing the human connection is the motivation, the pleasure, and the satisfaction of being a PT.

About the Author

Anne Ahlman was born in San Francisco but grew up on an airplane, traveling to more than thirty countries before her sixteenth birthday. Although she has never enjoyed the discomfort of long journeys, Anne developed a keen interest in the resilience of human nature on her travels around the world. Half British, she spent many holidays with her maternal family in northern England, where she first discovered her love of shared history, horses, and chocolate.

Always interested in the connection between kindred spirits, Anne was driven to abandon her career in medical research to pursue a more direct, personal way to help others. She obtained a master's degree from the UCSF/SFSU Graduate Programs in Physical Therapy, and has performed patient care in many settings, including acute care, orthopedics, sports medicine, hippotherapy, home health care, and geriatrics. Anne prefers the individualized approach to health care, seeking to reconcile meaningful functional activity with rehabilitation and wellness.

Anne has written numerous continuing education courses for health professionals, provided peer reviews, and published a variety of articles on health and medicine. She is currently the physical therapy editor of *Today in PT* magazine, a publication of Gannett Healthcare Group.

Anne and her husband Jim live in the San Francisco Bay Area with their cats Thomasina, Thistle, Koko, The Pie; and Atlas the horse.